I Wear the Scarlet H
A Memoir

Dawn Dravir

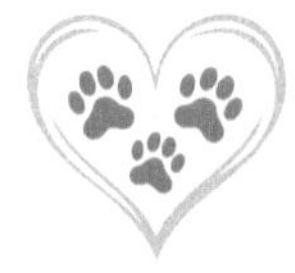

FRS Publishing

I Wear the Scarlet H

A Memoir

Copyright © 2026 by Dawn Dravir

All rights reserved.

ISBN (e-book): 979-8-9949263-0-7
ISBN (paperback)

Published by FRS Publishing

This is a work of nonfiction. Some names and identifying details have been changed to protect privacy.

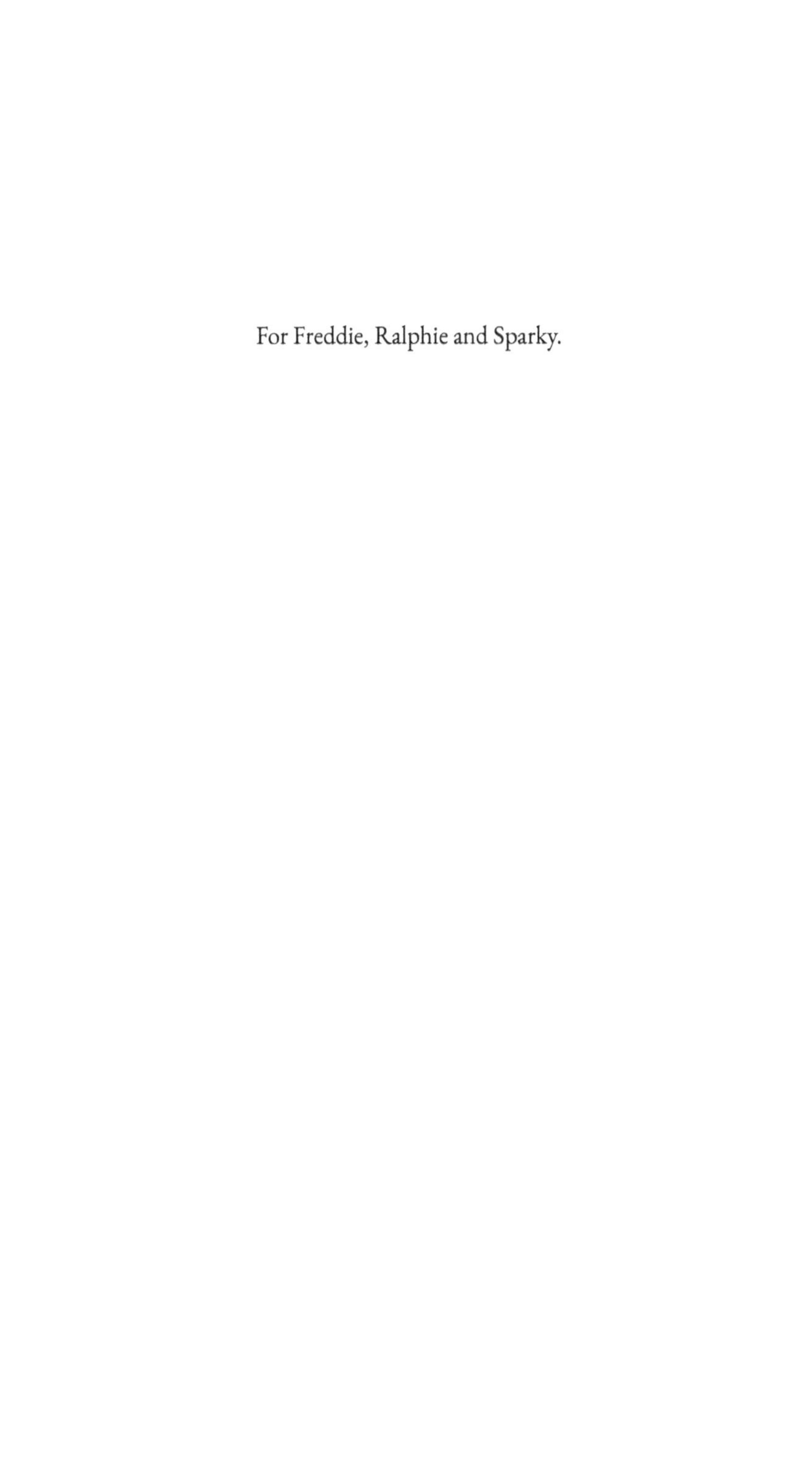

For Freddie, Ralphie and Sparky.

Contents

Part II - Depressed & Afraid

Part III - Acceptance

Introduction

When I was diagnosed with genital herpes at age 42, my world shattered—not because of the virus itself, but because of the crushing weight of its stigma. I attempted to avoid my diagnosis by revolving my life around the man who gave it to me, terrified of facing singledom with this "scarlet letter." Three years later, when we parted, I spiraled into a mental abyss, convinced no one would ever love me again. That fear trapped me in a self-made prison, robbing me of joy and freedom. This memoir is my raw account of clawing my way out of severe depression toward radical acceptance, a testament to the folly of letting stigma dictate our lives.

But let's dismantle the myths first. Herpes is astonishingly common, yet shrouded in unnecessary shame. According to the World Health Organization, about 3.7 billion people under 50—over half the global population—carry HSV1, the virus behind most oral herpes, also known as cold sores. HSV2, typically linked to genital infections, affects around 491 million people aged 15-49 worldwide, or about 13%.

In the U.S., the CDC reports that over 50% of adults have HSV1, and one in six people aged 14-49 live with HSV2. One support group I belong to states that as many as three out of every four people have one or both kinds of herpes. Shockingly, up to 80-90% of those infected are asymptomatic or unaware, meaning billions navigate life with the virus without issue. It's a skin condition, not a moral failing—manageable, often mild, and far from rare.

So, where did this disproportionate stigma originate? It wasn't always a scarlet letter. Before the 1970s, herpes was dismissed as a minor annoyance. But backlash to the sexual revolution of the 1960s and '70s, coupled with media hysteria in the late '70s and '80s, transformed it into a symbol of promiscuity's punishment. Time magazine's 1982 cover dubbed it "The New Scarlet Letter," amplifying fears amid rising conservatism. Pharmaceutical companies fueled the fire: the 1982 launch of acyclovir (Zovirax) required marketing herpes as a dire, incurable epidemic to drive sales, separating genital from oral herpes in public perception, when really cold sores can be transferred to the genitals via oral sex, and vice versa. Cultural judgments about sex and morality did the rest, turning a common virus into a source of profound isolation.

Through my story, I expose how this manufactured fear nearly destroyed me—and how I reclaimed my life. If you're battling similar shadows, know this: freedom awaits beyond the stigma. Let's rewrite the narrative together.

Part I - Submission to the Diagnosis

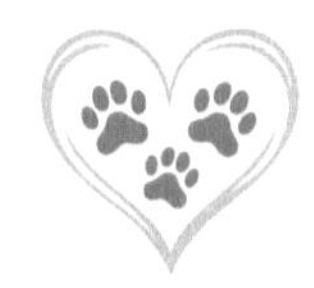

FRS Publishing

Chapter 1

Diagnosed

"*I have herpes. I have herpes. I have herpes,*" I repeated the words aloud to myself as I sat in my car outside Planned Parenthood, in August 2015, and wondered what had become of my life. From the driver's seat of my brand-new Kia Soul, I tried to comprehend if this diagnosis was now my reality. *Forty-two-year-old, healthy women who do hot yoga, have a new car, good job, no debt, and a master's degree don't get herpes*, I thought. They just don't.

I grabbed my cell phone from my purse, scrolled through my call log and found Ben's number. It was quicker to look in the call log than search for him in my list of contacts because the man called me nonstop and was listed repeatedly as an incoming call. My phone started to dial on my fancy car's Bluetooth.

"Heyyyyy . . ." he said, elongating the word. His tone was different, his confidence replaced with sheepishness, as if he was happy to hear from me, but also afraid to hear what I had to say about my little visit to this STD clinic.

I'd spent hours before the appointment consulting with Dr. Google and was pretty sure of my diagnosis before even stepping foot into the clinic. A quick care doctor two days earlier had told me he couldn't identify the red, irritated patches on my genitals. I was hoping for the same uncertainty from the Planned Parenthood doctor, although the knot in my stomach was telling me otherwise.

The morning of the quick care visit, I sat outside the building in my car for at least ten minutes before the facility opened. I wanted to be the first one in the door to avoid the chance of being overheard by other patients as I explained to the front desk person the reason I needed to see a doctor. But, as luck would have it, a woman with a sick kid beat me to the door.

I took a seat in the waiting room while the woman signed in with her son, who looked to be about five or six. A young, college-aged guy was working the front desk. I could hear everything the mother said to him and I knew she'd be able to hear me too.

When it was my turn to give the clerk my insurance card and explain the reason for my visit, I whispered that I was there for an STD check. I had to whisper the reason twice because he didn't hear me the first time. I avoided eye contact with the mother as I returned to my seat to wait my turn.

The quick care doctor was a handsome, short, chestnut-haired guy, who entered the exam room with his younger, portly female assistant. She had lovely, long, thick brown hair that I envied. I was hoping for a lady doctor because, any time a man performs a gynecological exam on a woman, a female practitioner of some sort must also be in the room to ensure the male doctor sticks to the examination and not any sexual perversions. So, instead of one set of eyes on your lady parts, a male doctor guarantees that there will be a second set to make sure he does nothing nefarious, but also to ensure that the female patient cannot file a lawsuit claiming that he had.

I hiked up the soft cotton white dress I was wearing, one of my favorites, and laid back on the exam table to let the two sets of eyes get a good look at my privates. As I lay there wondering if the heavy girl was feeling glad she wasn't me, I told myself, *at least I'm not overweight.*

According to the quick care doctor, the sores didn't look enough like herpes for him to make that diagnosis visually. I had used a razor and dry-shaved the day the burning sensation started, in anticipation of seeing Ben later that evening, and was praying that the redness was just a nasty case of irritation caused by shaving. The doctor said I'd need to have a culture taken to rule out herpes, *or rule it in*, I thought with dread, but he wasn't able to do that at his facility. He told me to make an appointment to see my gynecologist.

The doctor and assistant left me in the exam room to prepare myself to leave. I put my underwear back on and smoothed out my dress, which I'd worn that day in preparation for the local news to show up at the government agency I worked for. I thought the dress would look good on camera. Now this dress made me feel like an idiot in disguise; I was a deceitful person acting virginal in white when I should have been covered head to toe in black. I wondered if the doctor and assistant were in a back room laughing at me for being so stupid.

I'd just pulled out of the quick care parking lot when my phone rang. It was Ben. When the phone rang those days, it was always Ben. He called a lot and I didn't pick up every time; it was easier to just miss a call or two or three from him and catch up later. This time I did answer and gave him a brief rundown of my quick care visit.

I'd told Ben from the beginning that I thought I had razor burn. I didn't hide it. I considered it kind of funny that I injured my own groin area in an attempt to be ready for sex. When the rash got worse and I realized it was probably more than just razor burn, I still didn't keep it from Ben. He didn't appear worried that he was the source of my current issues nor that what was going on with my groin would affect his. He did seem puzzled by my attempt to get a diagnosis for what he was sure was a rash that would go away on its own.

At the time I thought it was sweet that he was unfazed by my rash, and I felt guilty that I could possibly have passed something on to him and caused him harm. Ben and I had only been dating for about a month and a half; before Ben, I'd briefly dated a man who turned out to be married. I wondered if that man could've given me something.

After dating the married guy, I'd asked my primary care doctor to order bloodwork and screening for STDs to make sure I was clean. After he placed the order, I noticed herpes was not included on the list of possible STDs and I asked why. He replied that herpes isn't part of a normal STD screening—UNLESS you have symptoms. I had no symptoms of any kind and my test results, for all the maladies I was tested for, came back negative.

In scouring the Internet, I'd learned that blood tests *can* determine the presence of the antibodies your body develops to fight the herpes virus. However, herpes is not included in a standard STD panel for two reasons: 1) the number of false positive (or negative) test results and the subsequent mental anguish carriers experience due to the stigma of a non-fatal virus that causes skin irritation and can't be cured, and 2) a culture sample from your body is the best way to determine if you indeed have the Scarlet H.

The quick care doctor advised me that diaper rash cream might relieve my soreness. I stopped at a pharmacy and, as soon as I got to work, made a beeline for the ladies' room and spread the cream all over. In seconds, I was in even greater agony; it burned like crazy. This wasn't razor burn, and a cream developed for babies' butts wasn't going to cure it.

I would've preferred to take a sick day to wallow in self-pity at home, but the 400 hours of sick time I'd amassed during my four years on the job—by being a healthy person who didn't get sick—would have to wait. This day was to be one of the most controversial in the history of the state agency I worked for, and our suite on the second floor was buzzing with excitement. One of my duties as outreach director was to talk to the media, and by the time I got into work, a few news vans were already parked outside.

The agency was on the brink of making a decision that could determine whether a burgeoning industry in Nevada would survive. The industry's PR team was far better at defending their position than we were; the online and media scrutiny was brutal. Every news outlet in town was covering this story, and I did on-camera interviews with at least two reporters that day. All the while my lady parts were burning.

Amidst the chaos, I was able to take a moment and attempt to make an appointment with my gynecologist. To my horror, I was told the next available appointment was well over a month away. According to the Internet, if I were indeed in the midst of a herpes outbreak, the rash would be long gone by then, with the average initial outbreak lasting no more than a week or two. I needed to see a doctor ASAP.

I'd already looked up Planned Parenthood a day or two earlier, when I'd contemplated going there instead of quick care to avoid having a second STD checkup in less than three months on my permanent medical record. But my medical provider's website assured me that quick care was an excellent place to go for an STD check, so off I went to quick care only to find out the website was wrong. I called Planned Parenthood and was able to get an appointment for the next day.

The TV cameras and protestors went away late that afternoon. My employer became the most talked about and hated government agency in the state for a while after that day because the industry in question died in Nevada and people lost jobs instantly. All I could think about was my crotch.

After work, I skipped my usual boot camp workout because my yoga pants irritated my groin area, which made it hard to jump around. Instead, I went to Ben's house, which was only a fifteen-minute drive from where I lived in North Las Vegas.

Because of my rash, I hadn't been to Ben's house in a few days, even though this was his week without his kids: Maddie, eleven, and Eli, fifteen. Ben also had a son, Tyler, nineteen, who was away at college in California. Even though Ben and I had established a pattern that we would be together whenever his kids were with their mother, he uncharacteristically hadn't pushed me to come to his place or to visit me at mine.

When I arrived at his house, he told me how pretty I looked in my dress and we watched my interviews on the 6 p.m. news. His friend and business partner, David, stopped over for a few minutes and Ben bragged about my interviews. He was being so kind, which made me feel so damn guilty! *What if I had given him a STD?*

After about an hour, I left and, rather than going straight home, stopped at Pizza Hut and got a large stuffed crust pie to help numb my feelings. Bingeing my way through my emotions was standard practice for me. I had two slices gone before I parked my car in my garage. The rest was gone soon after.

I loved the white dress I'd worn that day; it was slimming and showed off my toned shoulders. But I could never make myself wear it again. It hung in my closet for about a year before I got tired of seeing it and threw it away. I couldn't even donate it. It needed to be gone forever in the trash.

· · · · ● · ● · · ·

The next day, before I got in the car to go to Planned Parenthood, I summoned as much optimism as I possibly could. After I got there, as I lay on the exam table in the exam room, I willed, with every fiber of my being, for the doctor to tell me it was just a rash. I hoped the doctor would tell me to rest assured, that this was, in fact, just razor burn. However, that was not how my life was destined to turn out. As I lay on my back with my feet in stirrups, an elderly Black lady doctor looked between my legs and said, after just a quick glance, "It's definitely herpes."

My world was crushed.

I flinched in pain as she dug out a sample from one of the sores—there were three—and sent it to the lab for confirmation. At the front desk, I paid seventy-five dollars for a supply of Acyclovir and began taking the anti-viral medication on the spot. A few days later, the rash was gone. A week or two later, a letter from the Planned Parenthood lab confirmed what the doctor already told me—I tested positive for HSV2, or herpes simplex virus type 2.

My mind raced as I thought about never having used a condom with Ben: in my naive brain, I was safe with him because he was a father. *Fathers certainly wouldn't invite that kind of karma into their lives by intentionally giving someone herpes, right? What if karma were returned to him in the form of a deceitful person intentionally infecting his child, at some point during the child's adult life, with this scourge? And he wouldn't hurt a potential stepmom to his kids, would he?*

I'd waited four years after my divorce from my husband of eleven years to even try dating. Ben was only the second guy I'd been intimate with during my new dating life. The other guy I'd had sex with once, then found out he had a wife and two kids waiting for him at home. Several weeks later, I met Ben and started having the best sex of my life.

Before my appointment, I'd seen online that people experience their initial genital herpes outbreak within two to twenty days of exposure. After the diagnosis, everything came together in my mind and I knew damn well that Ben had given me herpes. Sitting outside the clinic in my car, talking to my new boyfriend through my car's handsfree Bluetooth connection, I felt like a fool for having worried, beforehand, that I might have given him some form of sexually transmitted ick.

"Do you have herpes?" I asked him bluntly and stayed quiet as I waited for his answer. I'd set aside all formalities, not bothering to ask how he was doing; I didn't care even the tiniest bit about his day at that point. I just wanted to know if he had herpes.

He hesitated for one second and said, in a matter-of-fact way, "Yes. But they don't know where it is in my body."

I had no idea what he meant by that and I knew he was making up a bullshit excuse to try and hide his guilt. I'd spent many hours scouring the web for herpes information and there was nothing about herpes taking up a mysterious location in the body. Even if you don't have symptoms or know you carry the virus - it's lips or groin!

"You could've told me!" The words burst out of my mouth with sorrow and pain and I started to cry.

I let the tears run down my face as I pulled my car into traffic to begin the twenty-minute ride from Planned Parenthood to my office. Still on the phone, Ben told me he wasn't worried about catching herpes from me, as if I was the one who'd brought the virus into our lives. He talked like a person who was innocent, despite the fact he'd just admitted he carried the virus. He said it was just a skin rash that wouldn't kill us. He would be worried, he said, if the herpes virus was a serious disease like HIV.

The damage was done. A life sentence was handed to me and there was no need to argue who gave whom what at that point. As I drove, I listened quietly to him over-explain the virus and the mystery of where the virus currently resided inside him.

Ben had honed negotiating skills, and they worked well on me, his clients, and the men who worked for him at his general contracting business. English wasn't his first language, and he didn't always speak it perfectly, but he got his point across and he always seemed to win.

I pulled into work, parked, and told him I had to go. After that, I stopped taking his calls and replying to his texts. I didn't need the words of the Great Steamroller pressuring me as I tried to come to terms with the reality of my life.

Meanwhile, a woman I'd known twenty-five years earlier, Jenny Johnson, kept entering my head. She had herpes too. Back then I was living with my big sister Doreen in the house she'd bought in downtown Somerset, our tiny hometown in western Wisconsin. Jenny rented a room from Doreen; I was nineteen, in college, and lived there rent-free. My sister, aged twenty, wanted me around for company, not to make money.

Jenny was younger than me and had just graduated high school. She didn't have a happy home life, which my sister and I were well aware of due to our friendships with Jenny's two older sisters, who were the same age as Doreen and me.

Jenny was already moved in when she told us of her recent diagnosis. The first guy she ever had sex with had given it to her. Instead of sympathizing, Doreen and I made her use her own soap bar in the shower and the toilet in the basement. We weren't about to catch her ick!

Everyone who knew Jenny knew she had herpes. Her way of dealing with her life sentence was to accept it, laugh about it, and tell everyone.

And everyone responded with disgust—even her family. The Internet was brand new and my sister and I didn't have the benefit of going online to search for answers to our herpes questions. But we had Sherry, Jenny's loud-mouthed and opinionated cousin, who showed up on our doorstep and read to us from a book about how contagious herpes was. According to the book, herpes could be transmitted from soap bars and toilet seats. I knew now, from my research, that this information was categorically false. I couldn't believe that I'd have to go through the rest of my life dealing with ignorant people who would shun me the way Sherry shunned her cousin.

Karma has a way of slapping you in the face. Years after not wanting to share a toilet seat with Jenny, I found myself in a relationship with Ben, unsure if he and I could have a future together, and I had become Jenny. From our friendship on Facebook, I knew that Jenny's life situation hadn't changed much over the years—she was still overweight, unattractive, underemployed, uneducated, and in stupid relationships with weird guys that she complained about all the time on her Facebook wall. *How could we now be the same?* I thought. The one way we would differ was in how many people would know of my diagnosis.

She told everyone; I ended up telling one person (other than Ben), instantly regretted it, and vowed to tell no one else.

In my misery, I confided my diagnosis to my co-worker, Jerry, my good friend and confidante. Jerry was an electrical engineer in his early thirties, married with a two-year-old son and another baby on the way. He was the least judgmental person I knew. Jerry was a trustworthy guy and, even though I didn't think he'd blab my horrendous secret to anyone, I immediately felt like I'd made a mistake. Feeling shame every time our paths crossed, I feared he imagined I was walking around with a continuous outbreak between my legs.

When I'd decided to try online dating, I'd gone to his office and asked him to take a few full-bodied pics of me to use in my profile. I'd read an online dating pro tip to include full-body photos because men assume, if a woman has only head shots, that she's hiding a fat body. I was an average weight, as I'd been all my life, and I figured it was best to be as transparent as possible.

Jerry and I laughed and joked as I posed for the stupid photos I needed to sell myself to a potential mate. We were an odd friendship – a middle-aged white lady and a younger Filipino guy. I could tell bits and pieces of my new dating life to certain people, such as my mom and sister, but to Jerry, who was so easygoing, I could tell everything. I texted him before dates to tell him where I was going so at least one person would know my whereabouts. And I texted him during and after dates to give him a rundown on how it was going.

I would've liked to have confided in my mom, sister, or closest friends, Heather and Nancy, but from them I seemed to get only judgment and warnings about the impending death waiting for me at each coffee date. All those women were also married and seemed to think I was better off single and unbothered by a man. I wanted to be bothered, and Jerry was unbothered by my tales of online dating.

Jerry happened to stop by my office the morning after my quick care visit and just after I'd returned from the bathroom with diaper rash cream burning up my crotch. I was miserable and dumped my tale of woe on him. As expected, he just listened supportively. I could tell he felt sorry for me. Maybe I even made him feel better about being married and out of the dirty dating pool with viruses and bacteria that could change your life forever.

After the Planned Parenthood visit, I could've lied and told Jerry the doctor saw nothing of concern, but I decided to be truthful. Judge Judy says often to litigants in her TV courtroom, if you tell the truth, you don't have to have a long memory, which are words I try to live by. And upon sharing the truth with Jerry, a wave of relief rushed over me at having been able to confide my ordeal to somebody. However, that feeling of relief was almost immediately replaced by a wave of regret.

Even though I knew Jerry wasn't a gossip and wouldn't share my secret, I feared that he could slip, and that telling one person would lead to my whole office knowing my shame. I'd have to quit rather than see the disgust in my coworkers' eyes every day. Would they sit by me in meetings? Would they be afraid to use the public bathroom for fear that I'd been in there and contaminated the toilet seats? Would they eat the food I brought to potlucks?

To protect myself, I decided Jerry would be the last person to whom I'd ever tell my secret. I also pulled back from our friendship because I felt shame every time I saw him. I wished I'd just kept my big mouth shut.

· · · ●· ● · · · ·

A few days after I cut off contact with Ben, I got a text from him when I was at work saying he was downstairs. I was caught off guard but went down to talk to him. Truthfully, I was touched that he'd made an effort to find me to talk things out. During my marriage to Leo, if I got quiet, he completely ignored me for days and weeks because, as he said repeatedly over the course of our marriage, "you got mad by yourself, you can get unmad by yourself." Our mutual silent treatments ended when I gave in.

Ben was there, of course, to negotiate. He told me that ghosting him was unacceptable and that I needed to talk to him if we were to continue our relationship.

I was mad at both of us for my current condition. I shouldn't have been so easy and gullible, and he should've been honest and given me a choice. I knew full well that if he'd told me he had herpes, I would've ended our relationship before it started. I'd put myself in this position of becoming what I viewed as untouchable by not asking questions until it was too late.

But there was also the possibility that if I'd asked about his STD history, he would've lied about it. During our first date, he'd boldly said to me that he never lied, which in my opinion is something only a liar would say. I hadn't seen any sores on his lips or crotch area, and I would've believed him if he'd said he was free of it.

Our conversation in the lobby of my office building ended with us thoroughly entrenched as a couple. I wasn't about to see what happened as a single person with herpes. Any reservations I'd had about him and my ability to tolerate his kids, who had become huge red flags in the short time we'd been dating, fell to the wayside. This guy was now my life and I had to do whatever it took to make the relationship work.

· · · ● · ● · · ·

In the weeks that followed, I became quietly obsessed with my diagnosis and herpes statistics. The genital version of the virus is very common, with as many as one in every four to six people having it. I got into the habit of entering a room and counting the number of people sitting around a meeting room table, at a restaurant, or working out beside me in a Pilates or bootcamp class, then I'd divide that number by four and six. If there were twenty people in a room, I'd tell myself that as many as five of them had genital herpes, or at a minimum, three. Up to 60 percent of herpes-positive people don't know they carry the virus. I knew I was one of the five (or three), and I'd look at others to see if I could guess who else was dirty like me and knew of their status or had it and didn't know.

I've read estimates that 50 to 90 percent of Americans have oral herpes, or cold sores on their lips. Oral herpes, also known as herpes simplex virus type 1, or HSV1, is easily spread from the lips to the privates. In fact, most new cases of genital herpes come from HSV1, whereas it's not as common to spread HSV2 (genital herpes) from the groin to the lips.

I'd look at everyone in that room of twenty people and calculate that ten to eighteen of them had a virus they could spread from their lips to their partner's penis or clitoris with oral sex. Who were they to judge me when they could effortlessly infect their sexual partners? At least I was taking an antiviral medication that made it extremely less likely that I could pass my curse on to other people, unlike these silent spreaders.

What was clear to me was that many people were hiding their status, just like I was. With the exception of Jenny, I knew of no one who spoke openly of having genital herpes. But it's a common condition! The fact I didn't know anyone who admitted having the virus meant that there were a lot of people out there in the world suffering in silence. *Those people keep silent for good reason*, I thought, which was probably to avoid the look of shame and disgust in the eyes of people around them. I would be like them and keep my life sentence between Ben and me.

Chapter 2
The First Date

One early evening in July, I sat in 100-degree heat on a bench outside California Pizza Kitchen waiting for an Israeli man to show up for a date. The Israeli, Ben, had suggested getting together a day earlier, on the 4th of July. I'd already made plans to hang out with my friend Heather and her family, and I wasn't about to change my plans with my longtime friend for a stranger.

I was forty-two years old and had decided to try online dating for the first time because I wasn't into the bar scene and I really knew no other way to meet a potential mate. Even if I'd wanted to go out drinking, I only had two real friends, Heather and Nancy, and neither one of them were going to join me in my man quest. Heather was a couple years younger than me, married with three kids under the age of ten. Nancy was in her mid-fifties, married to a man with lung cancer, and dealing with an adult, meth-addicted son.

Heather and Nancy were the first friends I made when Leo and I moved to Las Vegas in 2002 from San Francisco. The three of us met as coworkers at the health department, where they still worked. I'd moved on from there to the county building department, and from there I'd gone on to work for the state. Our scene was the buffet at the Cannery or Aliante casinos because we could sit for hours and chat and the wait staff didn't force us out. They were nice ladies and good friends, but they definitely weren't wingmen.

An acquaintance, Anisa, a chatty, rail-thin woman of Japanese and El Salvadorian descent, who I'd met at my hot yoga studio, had encouraged me to give online dating a try. She liked to talk about her Japanese heritage and time spent growing up in Japan but made hardly a mention of her Hispanic side. She was a year older than me, divorced with two young daughters, and had just recently entered the online dating scene herself. She made me feel better about taking to the Internet to find a man because she was an attractive lady, yet she needed the helping hand of the world wide web to date.

Anisa gave me pointers on how to set up my profile, what to write in my description, and how to get the most profile views with simple tricks, one of which was to change a word or two every couple weeks to trick the dating site's algorithm into thinking I'd updated my profile. According to her, updated profiles were given priority in being shown to men, and more views meant more likes and more opportunities for dates.

With Anisa's encouragement, I set up a profile and paid for a three-month subscription to Match.com. An ex-coworker I'd worked with at my county job, Thomas, unknowingly gave me my main strategy. It had been a few years since I'd last seen Thomas, but I remembered well the story of how he met his wife on the same site I'd just subscribed to.

Thomas was a chubby, bald, fifty-year-old civil engineer who'd claimed for years to be from Holland. He said fear of discrimination caused him to hide his true ethnicity and change his name to an ul-tra-white sounding first and last name. He'd only recently come out as a Palestinian who grew up in a Syrian refugee camp. To me it sounded like he had a speech impediment, not an accent, and it took me a while before I believed he was even foreign.

When Thomas was divorced, in his forties and in therapy, his therapist had suggested that he develop a list of criteria he was looking for in a partner and meet as many women as possible until he found the one with the most qualities on his list. Employing that strategy led Thomas to Millet, a fun-loving Filipino lady who had recently divorced her fuddy-duddy White-guy husband of nearly twenty-five years. Together Thomas and Millet held parties just for the heck of it. They decided on a whim at midnight to go see the sun rise over a California beach. They took trips together to see his family in Syria, who he hadn't seen since he came to the United States as a college student. And they took trips to the Philippines, where they'd eventually retire to enjoy the lower cost of living.

I didn't have any written criteria for my perfect man; I did usually gravitate toward guys with dark hair and dark eyes, though. Las Vegas is also a melting pot, and I found myself drawn to men with different ethnicities or cultures than mine. I love an accent.

My three-month membership to Match.com was set to expire in a month and I wasn't going to renew it. So far, I'd chatted with and met several men. My plan was to give up on Match when the three months was up and let nature decide whether I met a guy in my daily comings and goings. In the meantime, I figured it wouldn't hurt to try Thomas's strategy: meet as many guys as possible, weed out the incompatibles, and hopefully be left with the last man standing.

My goal in dating was mainly to find somebody to hang out with. I wasn't looking for marriage or a father for a late-in-life child. I'd achieved middle age without getting the itch to be a mother and I still didn't have it. I imagined myself spending a night or two each week with this boyfriend, at his house or mine, and going on occasional day or weekend trips to hiking trails or cool places in the desert southwest. As it turned out, dating was hard, time consuming, stressful, and oftentimes a real downer.

I wondered if maybe I was too picky. There was always something that turned me off. One guy worked for the city of Las Vegas, had a small head, and drove a scooter. I would've had to pick him up anytime we went further than a couple miles from his apartment. Another guy, a truck driver from Cuba, looked like he hadn't brushed his teeth in a while. The Cuban was able to make me laugh, but there was no way I was going to kiss that mouth. Another guy, with sandy brown hair and average-looking, was funny and open in his texts, but when we met, he wouldn't look me in the eye and didn't talk unless I asked him a question. I left him sitting in Starbucks.

The first guy who I felt sexually attracted to was a dark-haired guy from El Salvador. He was in the process of starting an insurance business and owned two homes. We almost had sex the first night we met in the backseat of my car, and then a couple weeks later he came over to my house and we did it. Then I found out he was married. I also found out he had anger issues, after I cut it off. He sent me a nasty text in which he told me I was white trash and all kinds of other sweet nothings about my race and unattractiveness. A couple days later he did a complete 180 and sent me another text calling me babe and asking to see each other again.

In those days, I knew my value and there was no way I was going to be disrespected and humiliated by a man. No way! I had a house, I had a good job with a pension, I had money in the bank, and I was educated. I'd gone to night school, earned a master's degree a few years earlier, and had no student debt or credit card debt. I stayed in decent shape and believed I was the master of my own life. I wasn't looking for anyone to take care of me. I wanted an equal, a friend and companion. I wanted someone to go to the movies with!

A couple days before my date with Ben, I'd had a drink and seen a movie with a guy who was a non-practicing Muslim from Egypt who owned commercial real estate property. We met for a drink at Blue Martini, and I had to hold off on taking a sip from my drink until my hands stopped shaking. I felt an immediate connection to this guy, which made me nervous. He'd been married to a white woman from Ohio, with whom he also had a young son, and as a white woman from Wisconsin, I was right up his alley. As an interesting foreigner and successful real estate investor, he was right up mine.

We ended up having such a nice time chatting and getting to know each other, he suggested keeping the evening going by seeing a movie in the theatre conveniently located across from Blue Martini. In the theatre, we kissed a little and it was nice. When we said good night, he asked if I'd like to go out again and I said yes. He would be only the second guy from Match who I'd agreed to see twice.

When it came time to meet Ben, I found it slightly amusing that I'd met an Arab Muslim a couple days earlier and now was about to meet an Israeli Jew; it was as if I was working my way around the Middle East! When I met the Egyptian, I already had the dates set up with Ben and felt no need to cancel just because we'd had one good date.

It was Ben's idea to meet at Downtown Summerlin, a new outdoor mall in the snazzy Summerlin master-planned community on the west side of Las Vegas. As I waited for my date, I looked around at all the fancy newness of the place and decided I probably wouldn't do much shopping here. Everything looked expensive—not necessarily out of my price range, but out of the range I was willing to pay for a shirt or a pair of pants.

I'm a casual, low-key type of gal and, for my dates, I dressed specifically to show that. I didn't wear short dresses, push-up bras, short shorts, or high heels. I didn't even own a pair of pumps. I didn't want to give my dates the first impression that I was a sexy or sophisticated dresser; it would've been too hard of an image to maintain. I like being casual; it's comfortable and takes little effort. The mid-thigh khaki shorts I was wearing, V-neck T-shirt, and sporty sandals would give exactly the impression I wanted.

I knew from the Israeli's profile photos that he resembled a tall, lanky, blond Canadian comedian named Ryan Stiles. He was not my type *at all*, but I'd also never met an Israeli and was intrigued. Even though I'd always had a thing for dark hair and eyes, I was committed not to turn down the opportunity to meet a fella based solely on his looks. Unless he was chubby. Chubby was a deal breaker for me.

I saw him walking toward the bench with a smile on his face and I felt a hint of nervousness overcome me; my hands started to shake a little. Our eyes met and I smiled back. I stood as he got closer and took a few steps in his direction. He was looking hard at me, and I felt a little uncomfortable.

"Ben?" I asked, even though I knew it was him.

We were standing only a few feet from each other, and I could tell that he was truly six feet tall. I learned from online dating experience that guys lie about their height and body type, which makes no sense because, when you meet, the truth will immediately come out. I'm 5'6", and if I'm standing nearly eye-to-eye with a person who says he's six feet tall, and his belly is sticking out of his supposed athletic body, it's an immediate "no" for me. I'll still go through with the drink or coffee just in case the personality outshines the lie, but that had generally not been the case. The whole time I was with one of the liars, I would wonder if he knew that I knew he was a liar, or if he'd successfully deluded himself into being tall and athletic in his own mind.

Ben held our eye contact, staring at me intently.

"You have beautiful eyes," he said with a cool accent that I liked immediately.

I do have pretty eyes. If he'd said I had a great ass, I would've doubted his sincerity. But I know my eyes are pretty. They're big and very blue, especially in the bright sunlight, which was the case at this moment.

He was dressed in a light blue polo shirt the color of the Star of David on the Israeli flag, and shiny jeans that looked almost like faux leather. They were kind of funny looking, and I knew without a doubt he didn't buy them in the US. My first impression was that he hadn't been in this country very long.

Up to that point our exchanges had been short and on text. He tried calling me once, but I didn't answer on purpose. I was uncomfortable talking on the phone with strangers; text was good enough for me. We hadn't planned what we were going to do at Downtown Summerlin once we got there, and now the decision had to be made. We agreed that we weren't hungry enough for a meal, so we decided to have a drink at a bar across the way called Public School 702, or PS 702.

The bar was on the second floor of an open-air building that had a street running through it. It was a ten-mile-per-hour road that led to other destinations within the mall and was blocked off every Saturday for a fancy farmers market where people from Utah and California sold honey and vegetables, and locals sold hummus, salsa, and arts and crafts. Ben was a few steps ahead of me on the escalator and I got a good look at his pants from behind. Even from this vantage point, I couldn't tell if they were faux leather or denim. They glistened in the light.

We took a seat in a booth outside on the patio. The weather was perfect; it was a typical desert summer night. The sun was setting and a nice breeze made sitting outside comfortable despite the heat. He ordered a Stella, the only beer he said he liked, and I had a margarita, on the rocks, with salt on the rim of the glass.

Our conversation was light and we chatted easily. I told him I used to work for a local building department, and we shared some laughs and gossip about people I used to work with and who he'd encountered through his general contracting business. It was a nice ice breaker that we knew some of the same people.

I recounted the highlights of my life, starting with my graduation from the University of Wisconsin, River Falls, with a degree in English and minors in French and Spanish. I told him about my plan, after graduation, to travel the world teaching adults English as a foreign language and writing. I would land in one country and write and teach until I got tired of that country, then move on to the next.

About a year into my Mexico experience, I'd admitted to myself that I hated teaching and there was no way it would take me further than Guadalajara. I over-prepared for all my classes and got nauseous before I had to stand in front of my students and explain English grammar. It was like being on stage performing, and I was no actor. Luckily, I'd met Leonardo, or Leo, and he became my excuse to give up on the dream of being a traveling writer financed by teaching.

Leo, who was studying to be a dentist, wanted to come to the United States to start a dental laboratory. He had a business partner lined up, a dentist for whom Leo provided dental technician services, and who was in the process of moving to California with his family. Leo just needed a way to meet him there.

We'd known each other three months by the time I left Mexico to return to the US. My grandmother was ill, I hated teaching, and it was time to go. The night before I was headed back to Wisconsin, Leo had invited me out to dinner. I could see the outline of what looked like a ring box in the front pocket of his jeans, although nothing was said about the box through dinner. When we got back to my apartment, we went into my bedroom and I sat on the bed. Standing a few feet in front of me, he took the box out of his pocket and tossed it at me. I opened it and saw a hideously huge cubic zirconia on a gold band. I asked him what the ring meant and he looked away in shy embarrassment. I asked if it meant that he wanted to be with me forever and he shrugged his shoulders in reply. From that moment on we were engaged.

Leo had wanted to get a tourist visa so he could move to the States and work, but that plan fell through when the US consulate denied his application. After that, I decided on my own to start the fiancé visa process to get Leo into the country legally as my intended husband.

Leo received his fiancé visa after I'd been back in Wisconsin for nine months and my grandmother had died. He flew to Wisconsin to meet my family in August, and a few days later we moved to San Francisco together. We got married at the Redwood City Courthouse within the allotted three months we had to keep Leo residing legally in the US. Even though we'd both developed many reservations about each other by that time, we got married anyway. I married Leo with the idea in my head that we could always divorce later if it became necessary.

After two and a half years of trying to figure out how we were to forge ahead in California, where it was so expensive to live, we agreed to move to Nevada. I'd read a newspaper article about the lower cost of living in Las Vegas, where even a casino valet could afford a home. We soon found out the article was true. Six months after moving to Las Vegas, we bought a house together, the house I was still living in, four years after our divorce.

Nevada also seemed like a more economical option for Leo to start a dental laboratory. He'd long since broken contact with his business partner and was slowly pinching pennies and saving to buy equipment for a dental lab of his own. I helped with ordering equipment, talking to vendors, picking up packages at delivery facilities, and getting permission from the city of North Las Vegas—including a zoning variance to operate a lab from home—to start his business. But there was one problem: Leo couldn't make the leap to quit his job and venture out on his own. He just didn't have the faith, tenacity, or fearlessness. So, after eleven years of fighting and still no business, we divorced in 2011.

I too did not possess the faith, tenacity, or fearlessness needed to follow my dream, which was to write a book. Instead, I focused on Leo's dream. Leo didn't ask me to work on laying the foundation for achieving his goals rather than my own, and I couldn't blame him for arriving at the end of our marriage no closer to being a writer than the day we met. But I could blame him for not becoming the entrepreneur he said he wanted to be and wasting my time.

Meanwhile, my marriage had also been sexless; that, I didn't divulge to my dates, including Ben. They didn't need to know that Leo and I averaged sex three or four times in a year. We fought about it all the time—I wanted it and he didn't. Leo said he was attracted to me, and his testosterone level checked out fine. He just preferred to masturbate—alone—to porn. Despite the fact that I caught him many times watching and masturbating to Internet porn, and that I'd discovered, at various times throughout our marriage, his DVD porn collection, his membership card to a porn store, and his browser history showing many porn sites, he refused to admit he had a porn addiction or that anything was wrong with our sex life. I was extremely lonely in my marriage; I also felt ugly and unattractive and feared how other men would perceive me.

Rather than get into the intimate details of life with Leo, I ended the synopsis of my marriage by telling Ben that it had been four years since my divorce and I finally felt ready to date.

Ben's divorce from his wife of eighteen years, an American with Israeli parents, had been a two-year battle that had just finally been settled. He said infidelity was the main reason for the divorce. It started after he'd urged his ex, Deborah, to attend her twenty-year high school reunion, and she begrudgingly did. At the reunion she reconnected with old friends, including an old high school flame, a non-Jewish mechanic who lived with his mother. She eventually started an affair with "Wrench Boy," as Ben called him, and was presently in a relationship with him until this very day. She also was about to finish studying for an online degree in family therapy and was in the process of changing careers from real estate to counseling and life coaching. We both snickered at the irony of a woman whose ambition was to help women and families in crises while simultaneously cheating on her husband and initiating a divorce.

He was an entrepreneur, a general contractor, who'd learned the trade while working for his father-in-law's real estate development company, where his ex-wife also worked. He'd started his own contracting business as a side gig years earlier for extra income. It became his fulltime endeavor after he was fired via an email from his father-in-law's secretary in the midst of the divorce battle. The wife's family tried to break him, he said, in the hope that he would return to Israel. But he stuck it out and was in the process of building his business.

He told me about his life in Israel, his time in the Israeli military, and how he'd met his wife and ended up in America, which he'd called home for more than twenty years. I'd been fooled by those pants! However, I was right that he didn't buy them in the US; rather, he'd picked them up on his most recent trip to Israel a few months before our date.

Not long after he and Deborah separated, he met a woman on JDate and moved her and her three small children into the home he'd just purchased as a single man. That relationship lasted six months. I listened in surprise as he detailed all the women he'd dated during the previous two years, including a second woman he'd moved in for a short time and a third who wanted to be his live-in companion. Two of the three had children of their own, and all three wanted to have his babies.

A current coworker of mine, John, has a theory that, after a breakup, the partner who has been scorned will try to find a new love as quickly as possible to prove to the world that he or she was not the problem in the old relationship. I one hundred percent believed Ben fit that theory, while I certainly did not.

We were on our second round of drinks, which we'd already been nursing for a while, and I felt like it was time to part ways for the evening. The sun had set and I had to work in the morning. I'd read dating advice that a couple's first meeting should be quick. So, I called the evening over after a couple hours had passed, even though Ben said he would have liked to stay out longer. He paid the tab and waved off my offer to contribute. Some guys didn't, which immediately turned me off.

Ben walked me to the parking garage where I'd left my car, despite the fact his truck was parked in a lot in the opposite direction. We continued to chat easily. He started to get into his ex's family a little more, talking about their wealth and ruthlessness. I could sense both his anger and sadness at the way his in-laws had treated him during the divorce and since. There was bitterness inside Ben and I wondered if he'd ever heard of the dating advice to avoid such topics on a first date.

I told him that I guessed I was lucky because I'd never met my ex-husband's family and there were, therefore, no in-laws to miss. Leo's mother died when he was three, and I never met his father, the stepmother he claimed was evil, or the three siblings he said he felt no familial connection to.

We were still on the topic of my ex-husband and the family I never met when we arrived at my car. For some reason, I opened up to this stranger and casually mentioned that my marriage had been sexless. We'd gone from staying in bed for twelve hours at a time and having sex repeatedly during the three months we courted in Mexico, to having sex a few times a year once he finally made it into the country.

Jokingly, I said, "Leo sexed his way into this country!"

Ben told me later that my comment about Leo using sex to convince me to bring him to America gave him the idea to move in for a kiss. He pressed my back against my Kia Soul with his body and started to kiss me with tongue. I wasn't expecting a public make-out session, and I felt weird, exposed, and uncomfortable.

A goodnight peck or short kiss would've sufficed on a first date. I pulled myself away because it seemed he had no intent on stopping. Turning my back to him and starting to open my car door, I said I had to go and was almost halfway in my car when I asked if I could give him a ride to his truck. It was an attempt to be kind, but I immediately regretted my offer. I hoped he wouldn't accept. He did.

He conveniently couldn't remember where he'd parked his truck, and it took a while driving around before he spotted it. He used the time to convince me to see him again the following night, a Tuesday, at my house. I was put off by his pushiness with the kissing, and now his pushiness with wanting to get together so soon after our first date, and at my house, no less! To make matters worse, I had the date with the Egyptian on Wednesday evening and I didn't want to be occupied three nights in a row.

Ben said his two youngest kids would be coming soon for their scheduled week with him and he wanted to get together before that. But I resisted. I'd heard from both men and women that finding a good companion in Las Vegas—someone with a stable career and no debt, no gambling or drug addiction, and no children—was exceedingly difficult. I had the upper hand, I thought, and this guy should be accommodating my schedule, not his.

As we pulled up alongside his truck, finally, I saw the magnetic sign on the driver-side door advertising his construction business. At least he wasn't lying about being a general contractor, I thought to myself. Or if it was a fib, he went to a lot of trouble to fabricate the story.

I told Ben that I planned to exercise after work, which was the truth. After my workout, he said he would come over. He pushed until I acquiesced, but at least he didn't try and kiss me again. I agreed that he could come over after my workout, even though I'd already decided I would cancel without ever texting him my address.

Chapter 3
The Second Date

The clock was just about to reach seven on Tuesday night and I waited with a mixture of anxiety and irritation for Ben to arrive at my front door. He'd put a full-court press on me all day with texts and phone calls to keep the plan for him to come over. He was persistent to the point that I caved and said yes. I knew I was being too accommodating to this man I barely knew, and I was angry at myself for not having a backbone and saying no.

I hadn't prepared anything to eat or drink for when Ben arrived; it was my little way of showing him that even though he'd convinced me to see him, I wasn't going to make him feel at home with snacks and drinks. Plus, I didn't know how long he planned to stay and laying out a spread might make him stay longer.

I had at least stuck to my guns and refused to waver from my normal routine of taking a fitness class after work. My usual routine after the workout would've been to shower at home and relax the rest of the evening in my jammies, with no makeup on and my hair un-styled. I have fine, shoulder length, mousey blonde hair that needs a round brush, blow dryer and hair spray for volume and lift. It's a fifteen- to twenty-minute endeavor that I prefer to do only once per day in the morning. But here I was, hair styled, face made up, waiting for a man to come to my house to do who knows what.

I had no idea what Ben thought was going to happen during this visit. Did he want to talk? Watch a movie or TV? I was definitely not in the mood for a make-out session, heavy petting, or nudity. And I wanted to be in bed—alone—by nine.

Ben texted "omw" and, after I googled those three letters and learned they meant "on my way," I knew that he'd be there soon. That text softened me a little about him coming over; I found it amusing that his second language was English and his text lingo was more current than mine. I figured having three kids—one preteen and two teens—helped in that respect.

According to Ben, we lived fairly close to each other. His home was north of mine, in the city of Las Vegas. Within the Las Vegas Valley, there are three cities—Las Vegas, North Las Vegas, and Henderson—with indistinguishable boundaries between them. North Las Vegas, also known somewhat derogatively as North Town to anyone who's been in the Valley for more than a minute, is the red-headed stepchild. Downtown North Town is old, grimy, and crime-ridden, and it was not a place I frequented unless I needed something from the city government. But the rest of North Town had varying levels of middle and upper class; it was respectable, to say the least.

When I described to locals where I lived in North Town, I'd always say north of Craig Road, or near Ann Road, as a reference to indicate that I didn't live in the ghetto. I was situated in a solidly middle-class neighborhood and my neighbors—Black, white, Hispanic, and Asian, were normal working schmucks like me. However, their children, from my experience, were assholes. My house had been broken into three times over the thirteen years I'd lived in it, and the cops said each time that the thieves were likely teenagers who lived nearby. The items the thieves routinely stole provided a clue to their profile; they'd kick in the front door or side garage door, run into the house, and grab small electronic devices, like cameras, tablets, and laptops, which they could easily hide in their backpacks from their parents and sell later at school. They were in and out of the house in minutes.

People often asked me if I felt safe in my North Town neighborhood. I'd say yes, but for full disclosure, I'd also mention the three break-ins, none of which left me feeling violated. It was more a sense of anger at having to pay the expense to fix another door and add another feature, such as a security door or alarm system, to make it harder for the juvenile delinquents to get in again. Despite the fact my break-ins didn't cause me fear, it confirmed the image of North Town in people's minds as a dangerous city where they'd never live. Still, I was proud of my little house, and I wasn't embarrassed to say I lived in North Las Vegas or that my home had been broken into.

The silver lining in Ben's visit was that he'd have the opportunity to see my house and know for a fact that I was self-sufficient and independent. I didn't know many single people, in general, who owned homes, especially women, and I'd held onto mine through my divorce and the Great Recession. I, unlike the other women he dated, had a home and wouldn't be begging to move into his, which I thought Ben would consider a bonus. Even if I never saw him again after this visit, I assumed that he'd feel about me the way I thought he should: I was a good catch.

The house was the only asset Leo and I shared during our marriage. Our credit cards, bank accounts, cars, and all other non-house-related possessions were separate. I argued at the start of our divorce filings that the house should stay with me because Leo got citizenship from our union and I had gotten nothing. The least he could do was give me the house we'd lived in since moving to the Las Vegas Valley in 2002.

Surprisingly, he agreed without a fight, although it wasn't due to my reasoning. The Great Recession had killed the home's value, and it was underwater by at least $50,000 the year we divorced, 2011. He was glad to be off the loan and his credit freed up to do whatever it was he was going to do, which turned out to be relocating to San Diego and moving into a rented bedroom in an elderly man's home.

Leo and I had accomplished our divorce without lawyers. Las Vegas is known for being an easy place to get married, but it's equally easy to get divorced. As was usual in our marriage, I took the lead and figured out what we needed to do to divorce as cheaply as possible. Luckily, there wasn't much for me to figure out; I'd already downloaded and filled out the DIY petition to divorce twice in years past, so I knew exactly where to go. The third time downloading and filling out the forms turned out to be the charm, as the saying goes.

I dropped off our signed documents at the Clark County Courthouse and did Leo a solid by paying every fee required during the process, which came out to about $500. Normally we'd split our joint expenses 50/50 even though he generally earned more money than me. Two weeks later, in July 2011, we were divorced.

It took longer to get Leo out of the house than to divorce him. He was slow to figure out the next stages in his life even though he'd had eleven years leading up to the divorce to decide what he was going to do after the inevitable end of our marriage. The country was still in the middle of the Great Recession and Leo's profession as a dental technician had become unstable. People put off getting crowns and bridges due to job insecurity, which led to Leo getting laid off from the lab where he'd worked since shortly after our move to Nevada. He'd always said his dream was to live near the ocean, so after four extra months of living in silence with me, he finally picked up and moved to San Diego.

As for me, North Las Vegas was going to be my home for the foreseeable future. A month after the divorce, I'd taken a job with the state of Nevada that paid better than my previous job with the building department, and I had a house that had tanked in value. I'd looked into comparable jobs in Minnesota and Wisconsin and found the starting salaries to be about half of what I was making. And I would've ruined my credit by short-selling or abandoning my house to foreclosure. Even though I was alone, with all my family in Wisconsin, Nevada provided a better living and I was going to stay.

Perhaps because I had no desire to date right after the divorce, I stayed in contact with Leo for a while. By the time he moved to San Diego, we were on speaking terms and I even went to visit him once. He also returned to Las Vegas for a weekend visit and we met once in Palm Springs for a few days. Even then our relationship was sexless and our friendship petered out after a short time.

Three years later the economy had improved and the Las Vegas lab where Leo had worked for nine years offered him his old job back, and he took it. He contacted me out of the blue to ask if he could live with me, and I let him move into my spare bedroom on a six-month trial basis. After only a few days, I knew it was a mistake. I asked Leo to find an apartment as soon as possible, but that stubborn Mexican was not about to leave until his six months were up. It didn't matter that we gave each other the silent treatment and passed each other as if the other didn't exist. Letting him move back in was a step backwards, and as soon as I got him out, I was only going to look forward. Looking forward needed to involve dating.

So here I was, sitting on my couch anxiously awaiting the arrival of the Israeli. When the doorbell finally rang, my heart skipped a beat and my two cats, who'd been lounging lazily in the living room without a care in the world, ran to safety under my bed in the master bedroom. I opened the door and there he was, more handsome than I remembered, in a tank top and jean shorts. His top, once again, was the color of the star of David on the Israeli flag. He sure liked that color.

"You look American," I told him as I looked him up and down with approval and a smile.

The expression on his face was of total confusion and he asked what I meant. I told him he'd looked kind of foreign in the shiny pants he was wearing the night before. My explanation did nothing to quell his confusion.

"I always dress this way," he said, referring to his current outfit and oblivious to the fact that his shiny pants were dorky for an American guy.

With that little discussion out of the way, I stepped aside to let him in.

After a brief hug, we went to the couch to sit. I wanted him to take a seat first so that I could position myself on the opposite end of the couch from him. But he was a gentleman and asked me to sit first. He sat close to me with about an inch of breathing space between us.

Before he got there, I'd been watching the news on TV and left it on after he arrived, which gave us something to talk about. Not that we needed it—our conversation flowed easily. We talked about the day we'd each had: my job, his business, his kids, and his parents' upcoming trip to America with another Israeli couple in a couple weeks. I would've enjoyed it more if it weren't for the fact that this guy kept trying to touch, hug, and kiss me.

He asked me why I pulled away from him. It wasn't that I didn't like him or didn't find him attractive; I'd already set my mind before he got there that his visit would be short. He'd pressured me into allowing him into my house and I was going to control what happened next.

"How are we going to know if we have chemistry if you won't let me kiss you?" he asked with sincerity.

From there, the negotiation was on. While Ben made his case for bonding on the couch, I mulled over my experience with the guy who'd turned out to be married. I allowed that relationship to happen too fast and I was determined not to be stupid going forward. But also, I'd already broken my years-long stretch of no sex by sleeping with someone other than my ex-husband. Nothing bad had happened to me physically; the bad part was finding out he was married.

Ben made a good point about chemistry and I agreed with his logic. I needed to be open to the fact that physical touch would most definitely be involved at some point with anyone I continued to see for more than one date. I also had to admit to myself that I found him attractive and interesting, so I allowed him to kiss me. I found it more enjoyable on my couch than in the public parking garage.

Before long, heavy petting was added to the mix. It felt good. After getting me aroused, he suggested we continue in my bedroom. I knew what would happen in there and I had no condoms, which I'd promised myself would be part of my sex life going forward. He told me not to worry because he had one in his truck. He ran outside to his vehicle and came back into the house with two. We both giggled at his obvious suggestion that he was going to get lucky twice. I liked that he could make me laugh, so I went with it.

We took our activity to my bedroom and proceeded to have fun sex, the kind of sex Leo and I had had when we first met. We had another go-around later, and then again in the morning. As a middle-aged woman, I thought the days of vigorous fun under the sheets were done, and I was pleasantly surprised—and happy to know—that I could make up for years of missed time with Leo.

The condoms lay untouched at the foot of the bed where Ben had originally placed them. Neither one of us mentioned them or insisted on their use. We joked in the morning that even if we had used the first two, we wouldn't have had enough for the third time.

As I got ready for work in my master bathroom, which was attached to the bedroom, Ben sprawled himself on my bed horizontally with his feet touching the ground and called his mom in Israel. I listened to the sound of Hebrew for the first time and found it beautiful. It wasn't just the language, but also the way Ben laughed as he chatted casually with his mother. Leo didn't have a good relationship with his family, which I theorized was part of the reason he was an unhappy, untrusting person. Ben's interaction with his mom made me smile.

I was smitten.

Chapter 4

It Could've Been the 4th

When Ben arrived at my front door for our third date, there were no pretenses about what we both wanted, and there was zero discussion about condoms. We went to my bedroom and had fun. And he was so much fun! We were both forty-two and rolling around my bed like a couple of twenty-year-olds. I never predicted what middle age had held in store for me: great sex with a guy like Ben!

I was still angry at Leo for having wasted what I'd thought were my prime sexual years on him. We married when I was twenty-seven and divorced when I was thirty-eight. Neither of us wanted kids and I was on birth control. We could've had sex anywhere, anytime, just to please ourselves, with no pressure to procreate or hurry to get dressed because the kids would be awake soon. I was there for the taking! I wanted it! But Leo wanted Internet porn and not me. Maybe Ben would be my reward for so many sexless years with Leo.

As Ben and I lay in my bed together, naked and cuddled up under the covers in comfortable silence, I wondered if the intense feelings that I had toward this man were love. It was only the third time I'd seen him. It was so soon, and I wasn't about to say anything about it. But then, as if reading my mind, he said it: "I love you."

"I love you, too!" I replied. All hesitation I'd felt just seconds prior were gone as I professed my love for a man whose kids' names I hadn't even yet committed to memory.

· · · · ● · ● · · · ·

I'd said those three magical words to Leo—*I love you*—just a month into our relationship, after concluding that since I missed him when he wasn't around, I must love him. The only other people I missed were family members, and I had no doubt I loved them.

I was twenty-five when I met Leo and had never had a steady boyfriend, much less been in love. Girls I knew in high school and college went through boyfriends all the time. Guys had liked me on occasion through high school and in my young adult life, but I generally didn't like them back. I remember being eager to spend time with Leo again so that I could share my feelings with him. The thought that I'd actually met a man and fallen in love was exciting!

When I told Leo that I loved him, also after sex, I was sure he'd say it back to me. It seemed to me that his interest was the same as mine. Instead, he winced. He didn't tell me he loved me that night, and I don't remember when he first said it, but I remember feeling stupid and wishing I'd kept quiet.

There hadn't been a slow progression into love with either Leo or Ben. Maybe this was how love happened to me—years of a dry spell followed by a relationship that came on fast and from out of nowhere. Within two dates Leo and I were already having sex, just like it was with Ben.

Even though there were red flags along the way to marrying Leo, I felt obligated to marry him. Without me, he couldn't stay in the country legally. Ben, on the other hand, already had citizenship thanks to his ex-wife, and there would be no feeling obligated to legally bind myself to him. We were just having fun and dating and could take things as slow as we wanted to. Ben and I hadn't even gone out for a proper dinner together yet. But I was looking forward to that, and many more days and evenings together with this man I could now say I loved.

I wondered, though, at the similarities between Ben and Leo beyond how fast we coupled. Both men were foreigners, although from very different countries. Both men had the entrepreneurial spirit, although Ben's business seemed to be providing him an income and Leo's business was mostly imaginary. Both men had August birthdays just a couple days apart. And the anniversary of our first dates was almost spot on. I'd met Leo on the 4th of July and Ben on the 5th, albeit years apart. I thought maybe the similarities were more than just coincidences. The kind of guy I gravitated toward was typically foreign, sexy, and motivated. But Ben appeared to be the "new and improved" version of Leo. Maybe the universe was sending me these similarities so that I'd know Ben was the guy for me.

Later on in our relationship, Ben would often say "our anniversary could have been the 4th, but you were busy." I always liked when he said that. I'd reply, "I would've canceled my plans, but I had no idea you'd become *my* Ben."

During our pillow talk on our third night together, I told Ben that I'd had a date set up with the Egyptian for this same evening. I texted to cancel that date, explaining that I'd met someone and wanted to see where it would go with him. The Egyptian was cool about it; he wished me luck and told me to keep his number in case it didn't work out with the guy who'd caught my attention.

Ben said he had a feeling that I was hesitant about him because there was someone else. According to him, he pushed so hard to see me the day after our first date because he needed to convince me to date him and only him. Despite how annoying I found his pushiness, I thought it sweet that he wanted to win me over before someone else did.

Ben also admitted that my story about Leo "sexing his way into this country" piqued his interest. He wanted a lady who was interested in sex, and my flippant comment made him think that I wasn't a cold fish. Years of a sexless marriage had ripped at my self-esteem and made me wonder if my female parts were even attractive. Ben assured me they were. That assurance went right to my heart and made me feel desirable. I told him that while my ex might've used sex to make it into the US, Ben had logic'ed his way into my pants with his talk on our second date about how we needed to see if we had chemistry. And I was happy he'd done so.

He told me about his recent relationships, saying his last three girl-friends had always been short on cash; he'd had to chip in to help out more than he liked. One still owed him money he'd lent her for rent, but he'd accepted he might never get it back. Two of them had kids who hadn't meshed well with his. Another was ten years younger and wanted to have four children with him. As a father of three already, siring four more was of no interest to him. I didn't have any offspring or want any; I owned a house, my income was stable, I lived close to him, and he liked my blue eyes. His ex-wife and all three ex-girlfriends had brown eyes. He was happy with all the changes I presented.

His last admission was that he had a five-year plan to marry again. He was two years into his five-year mission. I came from a marriage with a man who couldn't even propose to me and from whom I had to pull information throughout our marriage. Now I was with a guy who couldn't shut up about his thoughts, feelings, and plans, and I liked it.

Marriage wasn't a goal of mine. I was having fun and wasn't worried about putting time into this Israeli; I wanted to see where our relationship would go. And if it ended up going nowhere, I would be grateful for the experience and just fine going about my life on my own.

Chapter 5

The Routine

Ben was a lot of fun, but also very tiring. We quickly settled into a routine that involved being together at my house or his any day and night that he didn't have his kids. During the day he would call me as he drove from one job site to the next, which amounted to several calls, while I was at work, just to chat. I'd never had a relationship before in which the man put so much effort into me, both physically and mentally. He was needy and didn't like to be alone, and apparently, I filled that gap. My ex-husband had made me feel lonely and alone during our marriage and now my reward for the eleven years wasted, waiting for Leo to want me, was to enjoy being wanted.

Ben's oldest son, Tyler, was away at college in California and the younger two came to his house every other week per his custody arrangement with his ex-wife—one week with him, one week with her, plus Wednesdays with the non-custodial parent. When he didn't have custody of his kids, he had custody of me.

Ben had a lot of free time during his week without the kids. Sometimes he wouldn't need to be at his first project—usually a kitchen or bathroom remodel—until mid-morning, and he clung onto me until it was time for him to go to work. I was salaried and didn't have to punch a clock, so it was fine if I came in a little late from time to time. But with Ben I was late a lot, sometimes not sitting down at my desk until 10 a.m., and I worried my tardiness would catch up to me some day. I was an at-will employee who could be fired without explanation; I'd witnessed employees canned for less. I worried about repercussions, but I didn't speak up to Ben. Instead, I hoped nothing bad would happen with my job while I enjoyed myself with Ben and avoided hurting his feelings.

After weeks of this routine, my vagina was fatigued from too much sex. I'd never encountered this problem before and was tickled by it. Even though I was having a blast with Ben, I looked forward to the days he was busy with his kids so that I could rest a bit.

I would soon get another break when his mom and dad came for a visit from Israel. Ben had spent a lot of time with his family in Israel, where he'd been born and raised, while his separation and divorce were ongoing. His home country had been a safe haven for him while his marriage faltered and then ended. He said it had never been his plan to divorce his wife and live without his kids, and it had been hard to move on. He'd made mistakes traveling down the road to where he was at now— mostly with women—but he told me his luck was turning and he felt good. He'd just bought a house—the second one since separating from his wife; his divorce was finalized; his business was picking up; and he was dating a new girl with potential. He said he had a lot to be happy about and his parents' arrival topped the cake.

The parents would be in Vegas on Ben's birthday in early August. We'd only been dating a month and agreed that it wasn't long enough for me to meet his parents or kids just yet. I was gladly going to make myself scarce.

Ben had brought his first girlfriend to Israel to meet his parents—the woman from JDate who had three small children—six months after she and Ben met. She had a drinking problem and had embarrassed him in front of his family with her drunken antics; she had gotten angry because everybody spoke Hebrew and she didn't. Shortly thereafter, they broke up and she and her kids moved out of his house. This all happened within six months: moving her and her children into his house, taking her to Israel to meet his family, and then orchestrating the moveout after their split. The guy moved fast. I was content to move slowly in terms of meeting his loved ones. Ben's kids lived in Las Vegas and I could meet them anytime. The parents would return to Vegas someday and I'd meet them then.

Part of his plans while his parents were in town was to take them to the Grand Canyon. During the trip, he called and texted me when he could. One text was a shot of Ben and Tyler sitting outside their motel room smoking hookah, Tyler in a chair and Ben crouched next to him. Ben was shirtless and his hair freshly washed and combed. He looked so cute in that photo! I saved it as the profile pic for his contact info on my phone. Every time he called, that photo popped up and made me smile.

On the way back to Vegas, they got stuck in highway traffic just outside of Mesquite, a city about an hour and a half north of Las Vegas. Ben called me to ask if I could search on the Internet for a reason for the traffic jam. They'd apparently been sitting on the highway for some time, with no Internet service, and couldn't see a reason for the delay. I ended up texting an old co-worker from the building department who lived in Mesquite to find out what happened. Turned out to be a fatal accident a few miles from where they were stuck. Ben had me on speaker phone in his truck while I delivered the news about the accident. If the family didn't know about me before, at least they knew about me now.

Chapter 6
The Best Friend

On Ben's birthday, his parents took him and his kids to Outback Steakhouse for dinner. He'd picked Outback for his mother, who loved baby back ribs. Even though the ribs were pork and forbidden by the Jewish faith, they were also a must-have at least once when his parents visited the U.S.

I wasn't invited to Ben's birthday dinner, which was fine with me. Ben felt bad that I hadn't been included, but I assured him that I wasn't offended, which was a true statement. The only non-family members in attendance were Ben's best friend, David, and David's wife, Shuli, who'd been a late addition because David insisted on being part of the dinner. David and Shuli were Israeli and spoke Hebrew and fit in better with that group than I did at that point.

I'd met David and Shuli at a Friday night Shabbat dinner at their house a week before the Outback dinner. Introducing me to his friends was a good sign that Ben liked me enough to present me to peripheral people in his life and that our relationship was progressing just fine.

Until I met Ben, I hadn't heard of Shabbat dinner or its importance to people of the Jewish faith. From Ben's explanation, Shabbat dinner sounded like Sunday dinner, after church services, for Christians. Except in the Catholic version I knew, dinner was for immediate family only. My mom often had a Crock-Pot dinner waiting for us after church, or she made our favorite, chicken and dumplings, but the meal was just for our family of six. We didn't invite grandparents, aunts, uncles, or cousins for Sunday dinner. Shabbat, or at least Ben's version of Shabbat, was a dinner party meant to be spent with extended family and friends, an event he'd enjoyed while married and now missed as a single guy.

Ben was close to David, but he had no love for Shuli. He told me stories about her to prove that she had no redeeming qualities, except one—the man she'd married. Without David, Ben said, Shuli would be nothing. But even though Ben considered David a friend and enjoyed talking to him, he didn't trust David much either. I looked forward to meeting this couple to see if I'd feel the same as Ben or if I might find David and Shuli completely likeable.

Friday night came and I was sitting at a dinner table with David and Shuli, the people I'd heard so much about. I understood that Ben and David were connected by business, but given the lack of trust, I didn't understand the friendship charade and the need to share dinners and free time together. My feelings at that point didn't matter, though; Ben and I were just dating, not planning the rest of our lives together. And if we did stay together and become a couple, we could develop our own Shabbat traditions instead of dining with David and Shuli.

Even though Ben didn't like Shuli, he often complimented her cooking. He knew Shuli was skilled in the culinary arts, and Shuli knew it as well. Soon after arriving at their house for dinner, Shuli established for me, a woman she barely knew, just how much she knew about cooking.

"Because I cook!" she said to me a million times in explaining the depth of her self-taught, extensive knowledge of cooking. Her knowledge was so great, in fact, that she found it impossible to watch television cooking shows. Apparently, the TV chefs, including Martha Stewart, made too many mistakes while preparing any given dish. She couldn't tolerate their ineptitude!

Shuli was a pretty Israeli with long, thick, gorgeous black hair that I would have died for. I've always been disappointed in my fine blonde hair and I wondered how my life might've been different with a head of thick, luscious hair. I would've felt more confidant, I think, especially around men.

Shuli, who had an average figure and hadn't attended college, made sure I knew that she'd once been very skinny and was a top student in her high school class. She could've gone to college, she said, but chose to marry David instead.

David was born of Israeli parents in America. He was an ordinary-looking guy with big glasses, dark hair, and a soft body, his man boobs poking out underneath his golf shirt.

David told the story of how, while on vacation in Israel as a teenager, he'd met Shuli at a dance. He'd fallen so hard for her that he convinced his parents to sponsor her emigration, despite the fact she was a minor, to the United States to be with him. I laughed at this tale, thinking it was a joke, but then quickly apologized when I realized it was a true story. Somehow his parents and hers had agreed to the plan and, twenty years and three kids later, they were still together.

David wasn't shy about sharing details of his life, especially how he'd met and married his wife, the various businesses he'd started and sold throughout the years, and his current locksmith business. Ben said that David and Shuli were very wealthy and had millions of dollars in the bank. Their house didn't show as a home of millionaires. It was nice, though, with high-end touches in the kitchen—for the master chef, of course. It was way out of my price bracket.

Ben had brought every woman he dated, at least four, to David and Shuli's Shabbat table during the past two years. David and Shuli assured me that I was the best so far. I thanked them for their compliment and I believed them. I didn't have any of the other women's faults—no addictions or debt—nor did I have any attachments in the form of kids. And unlike the last woman Ben had brought to meet them just before me, an Israeli named Bina, I didn't argue with Shuli about cooking.

While dinner was delicious and everything went smoothly, I found David and Shuli's focus on themselves to be off-putting. Perhaps I was tainted by the warnings I'd received from Ben about this couple, but one thing was certain, despite their complimentary opinion of me, I didn't like them.

· · · · ●·●· ● · · ·

When Ben and I weren't together physically, we were often on the phone talking. Ben didn't like to text; he liked talking on the phone, especially as he drove from one worksite to another. I got used to wearing headphones at my desk at work and listening to him talk while I did various tasks. He'd tell me about the people in his life, his kids, his projects, his history, or any other topic that crossed his mind, including what shitheads David and Shuli were.

David and Ben's friendship had a long history that had begun after Ben settled in America twenty years earlier. Despite the comradery the men felt, Ben's ex-wife and Shuli didn't get along, which had caused a break in the husbands' friendship that wasn't mended until Ben's marriage was over. Through the Jewish gossip channels, David found out about the impending divorce and reached out to Ben in support. From there, Ben became a regular at David and Shuli's Friday night

Shabbat dinner table and David became part of Ben's plan to get his construction business up and running, the one he'd had as side hustle during his marriage.

David's role was to market Ben's company on the Internet in the form of search engine optimization, which he knew nothing about prior to taking on the task for Ben. He learned as he went and built several websites that linked to each other. One was a house painting website, another was for kitchen remodeling, another was for bathroom remodeling, and so on. The idea was, no matter what type of home remodel a person was looking for, they would find Ben. The websites were what Ben could see; according to David, he was doing all sorts of shenanigans on the backside of the websites to trick Google into displaying the sites in the top ten search results for home remodel in the Las Vegas area. Everyone else had to pay Google for such visibility, but David, a man who'd never created a website before, had figured out how to steal searchability, or so he claimed.

I was not impressed with his work; the websites were cluttered and old-fashioned, the content clearly written by someone with no mastery of the language. Each site was jumbled with photos, links to articles about home remodel, and glowing statements about how great and trustworthy Ben was. I performed webmaster duties for my employer and a nonprofit associated with my job so I knew a bit about websites; I didn't believe a word David said about his SEO prowess.

Ben saw nothing wrong with how his websites looked or the bullshit David spewed about tricking Google. All Ben cared about was getting phone calls from potential clients, and several were coming in weekly. Once he met the client in person, in their home, he would use his power of persuasion to help them visualize their dream remodel and, more importantly, sign a contract to start construction. It made sense to me that those phone calls would be his only concern, and it was none of my concern how Ben ran his business.

In exchange for helping Ben grow his clientele, David was to get 25 percent of all profits above a six-figure dollar amount agreed upon in writing, and Ben was to teach him the construction trade so that David, too, could earn a general contracting license someday. Ben's plan was to not show a profit above the contractual number—he wasn't about to give David a penny of his profits.

Perhaps David felt resistance from Ben. He began charging Ben $500 per month for his crappy websites and the mysterious online jujitsu he bragged about. Ben paid the money without flinching to keep David off his back.

As far as training David to be a general contractor, Ben had no intention of doing so; he didn't want to risk David stealing his clients. Overall, Ben was cordial to David face to face, but in private he'd often express his disgust for David; it made it hard for me to understand their friendship.

Chapter 7

His House & Mine

Ben's house was two stories, with four bedrooms and three bathrooms, a pool and jacuzzi in the backyard, and sparsely furnished. In the two years since he'd left his wife, this was the third home he'd lived in and the second he'd owned. I'd been stable in my house for thirteen years and couldn't imagine jumping from place to place like he had. At least the lack of furniture made his moving easier.

He had neighbors directly behind his property in two-story houses who could easily look into his backyard from their upstairs windows and see what was going on in the pool or jacuzzi. It wasn't an issue if you were just lounging in the water, but if you were naked having sex, it was a bit risqué, and I couldn't believe I allowed Ben to talk me into doing it in broad daylight. He liked sex and he liked doing it everywhere.

His house was about twice the size of my little house and in a relatively new development on the northern edge of Las Vegas. He'd moved into it a couple months before we met and had already made several upgrades to the property, including putting in large, glossy tile flooring downstairs, replacing the old kitchen countertops with new granite ones, and installing new carpet upstairs. I thought the master bathroom was already nice with double sinks, a separate walk-in shower and tub, and a large walk-in closet. If I lived in that house, I would've felt ritzy every time I walked into it! However, Ben had plans to modernize the shower and closet. Both looked modern to me in their current condition, and I had a hard time picturing what he'd do to make it better.

Despite all the things about his house that made it classier than mine, the thing I liked most about it was that he was putting time and effort into changing it into his style. He wasn't wasting any time making the changes either; I liked that. He wanted something and he went for it. He didn't sit around for years, like my ex-husband, thinking about things and planning for a change, yet somehow never getting around to doing it.

In the four years since my divorce, I'd slowly started updating my little three-bedroom, two-bath house. It was only twenty years old and still in good shape structurally. There had only been one owner before Leo and I bought it—a single guy who was apparently as cheap as my husband.

When we bought it, the kitchen floor and bathroom floors were covered in ugly linoleum, the walls were painted Navajo white, and the backyard was literally just dirt. I'd heard that Midwestern barns were painted red because it was the cheapest paint color available. It must've been the same with 1990s homebuilders in Southern Nevada and Navajo White because that paint color was everywhere, including in our house.

If I wanted to change anything in the house, Leo said I'd have to pay for it or physically do it myself because he was fine with it as it was. My attitude was that I wasn't going to invest my money into the house with no guaranteed return on my investment. If we'd sold the house, Leo would've gotten 50 percent of the profits without having contributed anything to the upgrades. But that deprived me of enjoying my home for the first nine years I lived in it. Just like our stale marriage, we lived in a stale house.

After Leo was out, I had ceramic tile that looked like wood planks installed in all rooms but the living room and bedrooms, which remained carpeted. I had a patio cover constructed off the back of the house so I could at least sit outside comfortably in the shade and get some use out of the backyard. I replaced the HVAC unit that broke down regularly with a modern, efficient model. And my mom and I painted the walls tan, with burgundy accent walls here and there. I regretted the burgundy color choice, but it was my house and I'd change the color when I felt ready.

It was important to Ben that each of his kids have their own bedroom. The second and third bedrooms in his house were furnished, each with a queen-sized bed and dresser, and the kids' stuff was strewn about in their respective rooms. The fourth bedroom, the one for the kid away at college, had just a twin-sized mattress on a flimsy metal frame that came free with the mattress, as well as two more twin-sized mattresses stacked against the wall.

Ben said the extra mattresses were to accommodate guests. He'd lay a mattress down on the floor in one of the kid's bedrooms if a friend stayed overnight or put both in the upstairs living room. It seemed odd to me, and kind of trashy, to keep extra mattresses stacked against a bedroom wall for the arrival of a guest once in a while. That's what couches were for! The mattress room felt unwelcoming to me, and I wondered what the college kid thought of sleeping in a room that was used for storage.

Soon after we became a couple, Ben took me along with him to a furniture store to look for a couch and love seat combo and entertainment center for his downstairs living room, which was bare. This furniture shopping trip would be our second shopping experience together. Our first was to a porn store located about halfway between both our houses in an old, white, concrete shopping center that housed three stores—two sex-related and the third, a tire store. The shopping center has since been demolished and replaced with a CarMax used car dealership, where I've also shopped for a car.

The sex shop had been a source of contention between Leo and me because it helped fuel his porn addiction. He had a membership to the store, which I found out about when he left his wallet unattended and I looked inside. The cheap asshole wouldn't spend a nickel on our house, but he'd gladly shell it out for porn.

Leo's interest in porn was something he kept to himself. I wasn't against porn and I didn't understand why he was so secretive about it. Hell, we could've used it to enhance our own sex life, which was mostly non-existent. I thought of Leo as I perused the vibrators and lubes with Ben and thought what a waste those eleven years had been. We could've had so much fun together if Leo hadn't been so weird.

Ben put his arm around my waist as we walked from his truck to the store and complimented me on my toned abdomen. He said I was the first woman he dated who had abs. My body was far from bikini-ready, and I had cellulite, but I also worked out and tried to maintain a decent weight. I walked into that porn store feeling like a champion!

On our second shopping excursion to the furniture store, he held my hand as we walked from the parking lot to the store entrance and as we walked around browsing the different options. My ex-husband hadn't been a hand holder and I wasn't used to being lead around in this manner. But Ben seemed to like me, and he had no inhibitions about showing that he liked me in public. And I liked that he liked me.

I was no stranger to the furniture store Ben and I shopped in for his formal living room; I'd been there years ago with Leo to buy a couch and recliner; it was the only furniture we purchased together. Everything else—nightstands, desks, TV stands, tables of any kind—I bought myself because Leo didn't think they were necessary. He liked the idea of a couch, though, because he was a napper and sofas provided him the perfect spot to doze off while he watched TV.

Ben had bought all his existing furniture at a different store—a store to which he could not return. He'd burned a bridge with the owner, an Israeli, after they'd haggled over price and delivery. No price was ever set with Ben—everything was negotiable. I sympathized with the store owner, as I'd already encountered Ben's formidable negotiating skills.

As we walked around and shopped, he asked my opinion about all the different furniture sets and eventually settled on modern furniture that was far from my style. I liked everything wood and warm, and he liked everything sleek, modern, and black.

The couch and loveseat he settled on were black leather and reclined electronically. It seemed like such a frivolous feature to press a button to slowly recline the couches, when it was faster just to use the lever and lean back. But Ben thought his kids would get a kick out of the electronic feature and paid the extra cost to be able to plug the couches into the wall.

Next, he bought a huge, black TV stand that was hideous in its modernness. Whatever this mass of material was made of was far from wood. It was shiny, ugly, and expensive, with two glass cases on either side. The price tag was also far more than I'd pay for a piece that looked plastic and manufactured in a factory rather than in a wood shop. But Ben loved it and called it "elegant."

There was no denying how different our decorating styles were. I liked the warmth and friendliness of wood and handmade quilts, and he liked everything modern, which to me was aggressive and cold. But

I also wasn't worried about this difference in taste because we were just dating. I had my own cozy house that I would continue to update in my style. I would live comfortably in my space and he would live comfortably in his. Besides, his couches were comfortable enough for sex. We broke them in soon after they were delivered.

Chapter 8
The Kids

I wasn't interested in partnering with a man who smoked, and I specified this preference on my dating site profile. If a guy messaged me through the dating site, I paid attention to his smoking status. Even social smokers—the types of guys who would bum a cigarette from a friend or stranger at a bar—were a no-go for me. I hate cigarettes. I don't understand smokers. I know that people do it for the buzz or to keep weight off, but overall, it's like telling the Universe you hate life so much that you're engaging in this avoidable, reversible habit to hurry up your death.

Ben's profile on Match said he was a non-smoker, so I was more than a little surprised when, a couple weeks into dating, he pulled out a pack of cigarettes and lit one up. Just in case I'd somehow missed that detail, I asked him what he put on his profile for smoking. He smirked and said that he noted I had no interest in smokers, which was apparently a common dislike of women on the dating sites, and he'd hid his dirty habit because of it.

We'd just sat down poolside to enjoy an evening coffee when he gave up his ruse as a non-smoker. Indulging in an evening cup of coffee and a cigarette was a ritual for him that I had, up until that point, been unaware of. The first time he asked me to join him for an evening cup of coffee, I turned him down for fear I'd never sleep if I consumed caffeine in the evening. He convinced me that most people aren't as sensitive to caffeine as they think and that I wasn't a caffeine victim either. He was right, the evening coffee had no effect on my sleep.

He preferred instant coffee to brewed, and his favorite brand was Elite, a kosher Israeli brand that came powdered rather than in crystals like Folgers. He heated up water in a teapot to make our two cups of coffee, sweetening his with artificial sugar and leaving mine straight, as requested. Shortly after we took our seats outside, he pulled out his cigarettes.

He wasn't a prolific smoker; he just had a few smokes each day. Still, I would've been a little embarrassed if my friends and family knew I was dating a smoker. And I would've lost respect for myself if I ever had to stand there waiting for him on a sidewalk, outside a restaurant or event, while he poisoned himself with those ridiculous disease-causing, disgusting cigarettes.

The fact that he smoked and lied about it were strikes against him when I considered the viability of a future with this guy. I didn't like the fact I'd been duped, nor the fact that he'd claimed he never lied. But I liked him. I thought he was fun and interesting. I had to consider that maybe I could be the positive change he needed to give up smoking at some point in the future if we were to stay together.

I had some misgivings: his weird best friend, the best friend's wife, and his deceit about his smoking habit were things I couldn't overlook. I already knew he was dating with the intent to get married, while I was dating with the intent to have fun. I liked that he was looking for long-term commitment, though, and I supposed meeting his kids would help me decide whether or not I could disregard the red flags that had already sprung up.

Before meeting his kids, Ben had provided me with enough information to give me a good idea of what to expect from each. I knew about their extracurricular activities and their characters. I knew Tyler was a popular kid who had lots of friends throughout his school career in Las Vegas and now at his California college. Eli was a good student, addicted to video games, who had gastrointestinal issues and had been bullied in elementary and middle school. And I knew the daughter was difficult.

Ben thought it would be best for me to meet Eli and Maddie at his home, on their turf. I would meet Tyler at a later date, when he was home from college. The day we met, Eli was playing a video game on his laptop at the kitchen table and we didn't talk much, but I came away feeling fine about the encounter. He was pleasant to me and seemed like a nice enough kid. The girl, however, was going to be a tough nut to crack. She was unfriendly to me and barely squeaked out the word "hi" in greeting, and that was only after being prodded by her father to acknowledge me. She didn't make eye contact and was adept at pretending I didn't exist. She spoke cordially and happily to her father and brother, but I was a ghost; she made sure I felt her lack of desire to know me.

I'd been warned by her father that she wasn't the nicest person when it came to meeting new people. I'd already decided my tactic would be to let her open up to me when she was ready. If Ben and I were to continue dating, I would be cordial, but I wouldn't try to engage her in any kind of meaningful conversation. If she saw my staying power over time, I reasoned, we'd become friends if I let the friendship happen organically. And if Ben and I broke up, then no time would've been wasted trying to form a relationship with this unfriendly child.

Maddie was slender and average-looking, with dark-rimmed glasses and straight, shoulder-length brown hair. She was into dance and theater, which I found curious; she didn't like to engage one-on-one with people but apparently could perform in front of strangers. However, I'd also heard more than a couple actors state in interviews that they liked acting because pretending to be somebody else helped them socialize despite their supposed shyness and social awkwardness.

Eli was as tall as his dad, slightly overweight and soft, no doubt from spending many hours on his computer and phone. He'd just turned fifteen and had no desire to work toward getting his driver's license in anticipation of turning sixteen. During this meeting and many other encounters to come, he wore black headphones with cat ears that protruded through his thick mop of dark brown hair. Ben didn't understand why Eli wanted such foolish-looking headphones, but he'd bought them for Eli because he'd asked for them. There was no way they were meant to be worn by a teenage boy; they made him look childish.

I was a quiet kid and could relate to Maddie's reluctance to associate with strange people. I clung to my mom at events until I felt comfortable enough to go off and play with other kids. Even as an adult I was quiet in a group, but after a few minutes, I could mingle with the best of them. Maddie was only eleven and I hoped she would grow into a more outgoing personality like I had. But there were huge differences in how Maddie and I were raised, and I wondered how those differences would affect the person she grew into.

For one thing, my parents hadn't gotten divorced during my childhood and were still together. They had their share of fights that my two brothers, my sister, and I witnessed, but they stayed married. There was no need to compensate for a divorce by overindulging bad behavior for fear the kids would choose one parent over the other. And for another, my parents believed in discipline and weren't afraid to employ it at the first sign of misbehavior.

After Ben separated from his wife and moved into his own place, he was forced to carry Maddie kicking and screaming to his car to take her to his place for his custodial visits. She was scared to leave her mother. As he carried her to his car, she screamed that she couldn't be apart from her mother because Deborah was her wizard and only her wizard could protect her.

Deborah was convinced that Maddie could see dead people. To help Maddie deal with her apparent fear of the spirits she saw, Deborah persuaded the girl that she was a wizard who would protect Maddie from evil. As long as Maddie's wizard was near, no spirit could harm her.

It took some time after the divorce before Maddie was comfortable visiting Ben without putting up a fight. I would've been scared, too, to leave my home if my head had been filled with the belief that only my wizard could protect me from unseen forces. I wondered if family therapy literature advised that teaching your child to believe you were a wizard was a good thing. It seemed harmful to me to put such belief into your child's head, even if your intentions were pure. The whole world outside of the home would seem scary to the child under those circumstances. Unless the mother's intent was to make the daughter never leave her, in which case, the mother was winning.

Ben blamed his daughter's behavior on his ex-wife. After meeting Maddie, I wondered how a woman who was a licensed family therapist could have such a weird kid. I felt sorry for the girl for the damage Ben said the ex-wife was doing, but I couldn't help but think Ben was also complicit in shaping his daughter's difficult and cold personality.

Everything I heard about Maddie from Ben and from what I'd witnessed was a massive red flag. As if smoking and weird friends weren't enough, that daughter was like a big, blinking, buzzing red warning light, telling me to abort the mission.

Further into our relationship, Ben and I talked about the role parents have in shaping a child's personality. I said that it was the parents' responsibility to mold their children's personality through discipline; kids like having some boundaries, it makes them feel more secure. Ben said discipline and correction for bad behavior weren't necessary, that the parent needed to step back to allow the kid to become who she or he naturally was to become. I liked my theory better because that's how I was raised—my parents made us accountable—and I felt pretty good about my childhood. And with his theory, you got a Maddie.

I don't remember much about my initial meeting with Ben's oldest son, Tyler, as it was soon after receiving the devastating news about my herpes diagnosis, when my head was inundated with shame, disgust, and fear about my future. He was tall and lanky, like Ben, and looked much younger than his eighteen years. He was cute, sociable, and pleasant.

There was at least potential to have a relationship with two of the three kids, and I hoped the third would lighten up after some time, because I wasn't going anywhere. Herpes was going to keep me moving forward with Ben despite any reservations I might have.

Within a few months of dating, Ben's smoking habit took care of itself. He lay down in bed one night and felt an incredible pain in his chest. He thought he was having a heart attack. Maybe the stress of his life had gotten to him and he had an anxiety attack, or maybe the well-known effect of smoking on the heart had caught up to him. Whatever the case, Ben quit smoking at that moment, which to me was a huge relief.

Just two more red flags to crush, the weird best friends and unfriendly kid, and we would be golden for life.

Chapter 9
His "First" Outbreak

"**I** have it now," Ben told me over the phone. At first, I thought that statement was meant to make me believe that I had herpes first and now he also had it. He seemed to be forgetting that he'd already told me he had it, despite not knowing "where it is" in his body. I listened quietly as he told me about his outbreak. This emersion of the herpes virus on his penis took place within weeks after my visit to Planned Parenthood. He said it was his first outbreak and that it was just as likely that I'd given it to him as it was that he'd given it to me.

Ben and I had been honest about our sexual histories, or at least I had been, and I assumed he'd been truthful also, as he wasn't shy about sharing tales of his sexual exploits. He had many stories of encounters with women from before his marriage, and after his divorce, he accumulated a litany of women to add to the list. Some of the women were from dating sites, some were tourists he picked up for one-night stands at a Las Vegas Strip casino he was fond of, and some were prostitutes.

Despite all the sex in his past, Ben claimed it was all protected—*except one time.* Just before I came along, he'd had a woman on speed dial for booty calls. For some reason, he chose her to have unprotected sex with. She wasn't attractive to him—she was just available.

It seemed unlikely to me that his sexual history was as consciously safe as he proclaimed. After all, he'd made no attempt to use either of the two condoms he procured from his truck the first night we slept together. But there was just no point in expressing my doubt that he'd always used condoms.

Since the time Ben told me early on in our relationship that he never lied, I'd heard him repeat that claim often. "I'm not lying. I never lie." He said this several times during conversations with me, friends, and clients. One time, when I caught him lying to a client, he told me it was okay to lie to customers because money and liability were involved. He was probably lying to me too about his consistent use of condoms—*except one time.*

When Ben suggested that either one of us was guilty of giving the virus to the other, I couldn't deny that there was a chance it had come from me. I'd had unprotected sex with the mother-fucking married guy from El Salvador. In the end, I decided there was no point in arguing over who was more guilty than the other. After all, this was the guy I was trying to make a life with because *WE* had herpes; I didn't want to know what my life would be like as a single person wearing the Scarlet H on my lapel. Nobody else would want me in this condition.

There was no need to be bitter or debate over who'd had it first; that would only lead to fighting. I had to preserve the peace to keep my life moving forward with Ben. Over and over, when I grew frustrated or angry about his kids, friends, or lack of time to pursue my own interests while we pursued his, I said to myself: "This is my life now." And I would acquiesce.

Chapter 10
This Is My Life Now

If I had to have herpes, I was at least relieved that I got it while dating Ben. I shivered contemplating what could've happened if the virus had emerged when I was dating the married El Salvadorian. He no doubt would've chosen his wife and children over me to avoid paying alimony and child support. As the saying goes, it's cheaper to keep her. I would've ended up alone, with no chance of finding a mate.

At least I ended up with the herpes curse while dating a guy I felt I loved, and Ben seemed committed to me. This settled my nerves about my future now that I was a pariah with an infectious disease that I thought would disgust even my closest friends. Would my two best friends, Heather and Nancy, let me use the toilets in their homes if they knew? Heather was the mother of three young kids, surely she would recoil at the thought of me using the bathroom her children used.

Yes, my herpes distressed me. But I was with Ben, and Ben was a lot of fun. He was a happy guy with a positive outlook on life. I knew he carried bitterness toward his ex-wife, and he was unhappy that his kids' lives were disrupted by having to switch houses every other week. However, despite these setbacks in his life, he whistled happily as he worked around his house, told silly jokes that would make you cringe, and laughed with me often.

After only three months of going back and forth to each other's places, Ben started planting the seed that I should consider moving into his house and renting mine. Whenever I was ready, he said, his door was open. I wasn't prepared for a step like that just yet, but I was happy he was ready, and I was confident that, at some point, we would attempt to live together.

Unlike my ex-husband, Ben cleaned, keeping everything tidy, and he was great at upkeep. If something needed fixing, he took the initiative to get it done. Plus, he was constantly thinking and planning on how he could improve things around the house. I found it attractive the way he maintained his place and thought that if I lived with him, at least I wouldn't have to worry about dealing with a busted electric socket or broken dishwasher.

During my marriage to Leo, I had to handle repairs because I was the native English speaker. But he would only split the bill if I consulted with him on everything. Typically, when I called the repair shop, the person answering the phone spoke with a Latino accent and likely spoke Spanish. So, he could've communicated with them fine. But no, he insisted that I call, and that I contact at least three companies for quotes. Then I had to take time off from work to meet the technicians at our house, while Leo went about his business with no care in the world. I took care of everything.

Leo was a procrastinator and Ben got stuff done. When our dishwasher broke and needed to be replaced, it took Leo forever before he installed the new one, which was the cheapest one Home Depot had to offer, of course. It wasn't that he lacked the time to do work around the house; he just wouldn't do anything until he was ready. And if I irritated him by asking him to please get to it, he would procrastinate even longer. Meanwhile I'd quietly stew and wonder how I'd ended up with such an obstinate man and if I could endure much more of our marriage.

Nothing sat undone at Ben's house for long and I liked that. Even a burnt-out lightbulb was replaced right away. I typically keep things in good condition but even I drag on such things.

Every other Sunday, before his kids would come back to his house for their weekly visits, he'd wash their sheets and clothes, put all of it back in place, and mop and vacuum in preparation for their arrival. He was conscientious about his pantry and kept it stocked with snacks for the kids. I accompanied him on Sunday shopping trips to buy food for them. He wasn't an experienced cook, but with guidance from his mother after his divorce, he learned to make a couple of his kids' favorite meals.

He was thoughtful in what he bought and prepared for them but not concerned about the healthfulness of the food. He believed that if a parent restricted kids from eating what they wanted the moment they wanted it, they would respond by eating more junk food in secret. He had a chubby son, Eli, so I didn't quite believe his theory. But it wasn't my place to say anything because these were not my kids.

From what I could see, he wasn't looking for a mother for his kids; he had their needs handled. In fact, the Israeli woman, Bina, who lived with him for a month just prior to my arrival, had tried to be a mother to them, and that was her downfall. She attempted to teach them manners and make them accountable for the messes they created in the house. On one occasion, she took away Maddie's phone charger because Maddie left her backpack sitting on the dining room floor rather than putting it in her room, as Bina had repeatedly asked her to do. Unfortunately for Bina, she might as well have been trying to get the neighbor kids in line.

Bina was ten years younger than Ben and was best friends with his younger sister back in Israel. She wore glasses and had a wonky eye that was either lazy or blind, but she also had nice, thick, wavy brown hair. She wanted to have four babies with Ben, which he let her believe might happen, even though he was disinclined to have more kids.

Ben had brought Bina over from Israel for a two-month trial run that failed within the first few weeks. The two had actually met in Las Vegas several years earlier, when Bina attended Tyler's bar mitzvah, having gotten an invitation through Ben's sister.

Ben was still married to Deborah at the time, but Bina later told him that it was love at first sight when he picked her up at the airport in the Hummer he drove until he was forced to sell it during the divorce. Bina had to bide her time until fortune would lead to Ben's divorce and their chance reconnection during one of his post-separation trips to Israel. They had had sex during that trip, and her performance must have been good enough that Ben wanted to see how they would do as a couple in the U.S.

Ben had moved into his current house shortly before Bina came over to try living with him. She helped pick out the dinnerware they'd need for the large Shabbat dinners they both envisioned; there were enough plates and silverware to serve at least twenty people. In her short time in Vegas, she proved her culinary abilities by cooking daily for Ben and his kids, and together they'd hosted a small Shabbat dinner for a few of Ben's friends, including David and Shuli.

Bina would've made a great Jewish-Israeli wife. She knew the traditions; she liked the large Shabbat dinners Ben had enjoyed so much in the past. But for the fact that she tried to install household rules for his kids to follow, she'd be living the life she dreamed of, with the man she had fallen in love with years before. However, his kids didn't like her and that was the end of her story with Ben.

And that was where I was at with this man with whom I shared the herpes virus. I loved him. I enjoyed doing activities with him. But his kids . . . I just didn't like his kids. And from what I could tell, they didn't like me either.

Chapter 11
The Cupcake

One typical Saturday, a warm fall afternoon in Vegas, Ben, Eli, and I filed into the middle row of the auditorium at the private theatre where Maddie had trained to be an actor; we were there to see her in a musical production *of Horton Hears a Who* by Dr. Seuss. My relationship—or non-relationship—with Maddie remained frosty, but Ben wanted me there, so of course I went.

I had never read this Dr. Seuss classic and was unfamiliar with the plot. After sitting through the performance by Maddie and a bunch of other middle schoolers singing and dancing, I still had no clue to the book's contents. I couldn't even tell, based on the costume worn by the boy who was the main character, that Horton was an elephant.

Maddie played the part of some kind of bird. There were three girls, including Maddie, whose costumes were bird-like. The three came out from time to time during the play as a trio and sang off-key and danced. It was obvious that Maddie was the only one among the three who had any dance experience, although the dance moves weren't complicated or extravagant and no dance experience was required to perform them.

It was odd to see that unpleasant little girl on stage performing in a sweet children's musical. I doubt that anybody in the audience would've believed that not long before this performance, she sat in a chair next to her dad, at David and Shuli's Shabbat dinner table, with her face buried in Ben's shoulder, a pout on her face. She refused to eat anything, look at anybody, or utter a word in response to attempts to talk to her. She didn't want to be at that dinner and was determined to make the evening miserable for all those involved.

David and Shuli also had an eleven-year-old daughter, who was a pretty and pleasant child named after a sports car, and who could hold a conversation with an adult. Although David and Shuli were braggarts who could make your eyes roll back in your head with tales of their accomplishments, I liked their daughter. Maddie did not. Those girls could easily have been friends and spent much of the evening doing girl things in Maserati's bedroom. But instead, Maddie chose to be a little brat. I was embarrassed for her, and for Ben.

Ben didn't give in to Maddie's attempt to force an early retreat home, which was what she wanted. But he didn't try to stop her from acting in an ill-mannered and insolent way, and there was also no punishment for her behavior afterward. There was no grounding of any sort, and not even the slightest of lectures. I couldn't imagine either of my parents allowing any of their four kids to act like Maddie without some sort of well-deserved consequence.

Once the dinner was over and we were all back home at Ben's place, Maddie returned to being her usual self. She was personable to Ben and Eli and only I was ignored. Ben let her raid the pantry for her dinner. She took the snacks she wanted and went to her bedroom. Her world had returned to her normal and she was content.

•••••••••

The boys at least tolerated me and were friendly. In late August, just after Ben and I had started dating and I got my herpes diagnosis, I accompanied Ben on a road trip to take his eldest son, Tyler, back to his central California university prior to the start of his sophomore year. I felt a bit like an interloper invading on this father-son time, but Ben wanted me along on this trip to keep him company in his hotel room at night and during the drive back home. Tyler didn't seem to mind that I tagged along, and he was a pleasant person to be around despite the fact I truly was, at this point, just another of his dad's post-divorce girlfriends.

Among Ben's kids, Maddie was the weirdo, Eli was the soft computer nerd and know-it-all, and Tyler was the extroverted know-it-all. Tyler was a born leader who liked to organize events for his fraternity and friends. He had a confidence he hadn't yet earned.

A couple years into our relationship, when we were all out having a steak dinner, Tyler and Ben were talking about the daughter of a family friend who had just graduated dental school and whose father had invested in the equipment required to help her start her practice. Tyler was expounding on the money that would start pouring into the woman's dental business on day one. Ben was expounding on the college and equipment debt that would take years to pay off. Tyler's response was to tell his father, with exasperation and contempt, that Ben "knew nothing about business." This, from a boy who didn't have to work a day in his life to pay for his college existence, who lived a life of ease and fun, who had no work or business experience himself.

Ben lowered his gaze and silently took this insult, and I bit my tongue. I wanted so bad to come to Ben's defense and remind Tyler that his parents were spending a lot of money to send him to college to earn a degree in construction management so that Tyler could do the same type of work his father did, on the daily, with knowledge learned on the job. But I didn't have the type of standing in this family in which I could speak my mind to the kids when they acted stupid. Ben wanted it that way. I really didn't want to be a disciplinarian, either, even though I often wanted to step in when I felt the kids needed to be put in their place, such as this time, when Tyler was talking down to his dad.

When Tyler had announced, during his sophomore year of college, that it was time for his parents to buy him a car, I wasn't surprised that he got it. He would've had a car already if he'd taken care of the brand-new Ford Escape his parents bought him while in high school. Instead, he trashed it. Among the many things he did to bring about the Ford's early demise, the final straw was a trip into the desert, in which Tyler treated the Escape as if it were a dune buggy.

I was in my thirties when I bought my first brand-new car, a PT Cruiser, that I paid off over the course of a few years. Tyler got a new car at sixteen that was paid for by his parents. There was no way, if I were his parent, that I would've even considered buying that child another car—used or new—after he destroyed the first one I'd bought for him. So, when Ben suggested, just a few months into our relationship, that he and I buy a car together, my immediate answer was no. I feared what he would allow his kids to do to it.

Ben had floated the idea one night when we were out on a walk; he said he wanted to buy a convertible sports car to replace a similar vehicle he'd had to sell during the divorce and suggested we buy it together as our first joint purchase. It would serve as the start of us merging our lives together, he said. I asked if his kids would be allowed to drive it, to which he replied yes. I told him that there had been no repercussions after Tyler destroyed the Ford and I feared that he'd have no respect for any car Ben and I shared.

My actual thought about buying a car with Ben was *no fucking way*. There was no way I was going to allow that kid, or Ben's other kids, to destroy any property of mine. I'd already experienced the disrespect his kids showed toward my Kia Soul, and I knew they'd show no care toward a sports car because they simply didn't have to.

. . . . ● . ● . . . .

After the *Horton Hears a Who* performance, I'd taken Ben, Maddie, and Eli home in my Kia. Ben was a believer in the idea that if his kids saw me participating in their lives, they would accept me and we'd all be one happy family. If they saw me buy movie tickets for everyone, they'd see I wasn't just taking from their dad. They'd see that I cared and would accept me. If they saw me drive the family to restaurants and other events, they'd see that I cared and would accept me. If I went to their performances and sports activities, they'd see that I cared and would accept me.

I don't know why the kids couldn't have been told to just be nice to me, but supposedly all this participation was going to show them that I was in for the long haul and that I cared. As usual, Maddie didn't acknowledge my existence at her performance and I sure as heck didn't receive a thank you for attending. However, once the show was over, she quietly waited to say goodbye to the director, a waifish White man in his thirties, while he finished talking to a line of parents and actors. I thought to myself, *so she can acknowledge people outside of her family, just not the women her father dates.*

I knew I wasn't the only woman in Ben's past she treated that way; Bina, the Israeli woman who came before me, and Anna, the woman who came before her, were both on the receiving end of Maddie's disrespect. Anna, who was half Filipino and half White, was a few years older than Ben and he referred to her as his cougar. Her attributes were that she was pretty and liked anal sex and asked for it. Her downfalls were her inability to pay her rent, her drinking, and her twelve-year-old daughter, Jenna.

When Anna and Jenna visited Ben at his home, Eli and Maddie responded by locking themselves together in one of their bedrooms. After Anna started hinting that Ben's four-bedroom house would accommodate her and Jenna, Ben ended it. She still owed him money for funds he loaned her for rent.

Maddie's rejection of me hurt only a little less when I learned that she was an asshole to all the women who came before me. I didn't know if those women had herpes or not, but I did and I wasn't going anywhere. I wanted rules, though. I wanted the kids to be taught to respect me. A stupid cupcake offered me the chance to tell Ben he needed to discipline his kids.

Each of the child actors in the *Horton Hears a Who* musical were given an oversized, heavily frosted cupcake after their performance was over. I had a feeling that cupcake was going to end up all over the back seat of my car, but I felt unable to ask Maddie to be careful because Ben had made it known I was not to be an authoritarian to his kids. I knew what had happened to Bina.

I took the driver seat, Ben sat in the passenger seat next to me, Maddie sat behind him in the back, and Eli sat directly behind me. The whole trip home, Eli and Maddie argued and slapped each other, with not a word said by either adult in the car to stop their actions and to warn them to be careful with that damn cupcake. It wasn't Ben's nature to tell the kids to knock it off, and I quietly stewed at my inability to tell them to respect my shit. I knew bits of the cupcake would go everywhere in my clean, new car, and I was right.

I pulled up to the curb outside of Ben's house and parked. Eli and Maddie opened their doors immediately and trotted into the house. I took a look at the backseat and saw cupcake and frosting all over the seat and floor. I angrily asked Ben why he couldn't tell his kids to quit their fighting; he had to have known that there would be cupcake everywhere.

According to him, his kids were allowed to destroy the vehicles he and his ex-wife owned. He justified their actions by saying they were kids and that's what kids did. But I wasn't their parent—why did they feel it was okay to destroy my property? And why wasn't he going to punish them? If they were my kids, I would've had both come outside and clean out the cupcake from the car. And no half-assed job either. Rather than disturb his kids from their leisure inside the house, Ben got his shop vac and a rag and cleaned out the backseat.

So, when he suggested we buy a car together to start merging our lives, I politely declined. I told him it would be best for him to buy the car on his own. He did just that and the kids drove it whenever they wanted.

Chapter 12
Nine Months Later

I texted my mom a photo of a little glass bird sculpture she'd gifted me; it was sitting nicely on top of the small, round wicker table that went with my outdoor wicker chair set.

"Guess where your birds are at?" I typed into my phone. I sent the photo to show her that the birds and my outdoor furniture had been moved from my back patio to a different yard.

The sculpture, four inches long and two inches high, consisted of two little pink birds sitting on a light brown tree branch. My mom had bought it for me at a neighbor's garage sale during one of her visits, despite the fact that I'd forbade her from bringing any junk from the sale into my house. I am not a fan of garage sales or thrift stores, while my mom will find a place in her home or yard for any used item that catches her eye. I did not inherit that trait. I prefer decorating with meaningful items that belonged to a relative or that were handmade and sold at a craft fair; I have no interest in random items from China snagged secondhand from a sidewalk foldout table.

It happened when my mom had walked herself alone down the block to the neighbor's. She thought she was being funny by bringing me that knickknack. I had the last laugh, though, by holding onto it and taking it to Ben's.

She didn't reply to my text. I knew she was upset that I'd taken the plunge and moved in with Ben. She'd told me that moving in with him shouldn't even be up for debate at this early stage in our relationship, and I had no doubt that she was right. But she also didn't know that I had herpes, and in my mind, I was going to spend the rest of my days with this man, so there was no reason to put off the inevitable. Besides, I had a house and could move back into it if living with Ben and his kids took a turn for the worse.

My mom had been a frequent guest at my home in North Las Vegas before my divorce, and she became an even more frequent guest after there was no longer a sullen Mexican in the house making her and other family members feel unwelcome during their stays. Moving in with Ben didn't fit into her retirement plan of avoiding Wisconsin winters by staying with me in Nevada during the coldest months of the year. She made it clear that she would not visit me if I lived with Ben; she just wouldn't feel comfortable around his kids.

I complained a lot to my friends and loved ones about Maddie, Eli, and Tyler. A LOT. I knew I didn't paint a flattering picture of the kids, and my mom had no desire to receive the same treatment I complained about ALL THE TIME. But I also wanted my family and friends to meet them because I was sure their impressions would match mine and I could prove to Ben that he needed to require change from his children.

My mom had met Ben and was comfortable around him, even though she and the rest of my family couldn't quite see what had attracted me to him. He was the opposite of my ex-husband in so many ways, including the ease with which he held a conversation with people and the way he looked. Leo was short and dark; Ben was tall, dirty blond, and White, owing to his Polish ancestry.

Ben accompanied me on a Christmas trip to Wisconsin after we'd been together just five months and, for the most part, got along well with my family. The exception was that my sister thought he was too controlling of me, and I could see the annoyance on my brother Tim's face as Ben bragged about the Hummer and other possessions he'd once owned but had to sell due to his divorce. And he didn't ingratiate himself with my family by making suggestions on how to improve the peaceful Wisconsin they loved by building storage units and quick care facilities in fields. He also made suggestions on how they could improve their practical living spaces with room additions and remodels. He saw unutilized space everywhere and wondered why people who owned several acres didn't take advantage of their land by building bigger houses. My people saw a city slicker who wanted to ruin their rural lifestyle and they didn't like it. But despite the hurt some of his opinions caused and his pushiness towards me, it was a decent trip, and my family made an effort to like Ben because I liked him.

I hated taking Leo to visit my family in Wisconsin. He was always bored, and it was stressful for me to keep him entertained. He didn't like interacting with people and would often sneak off to take naps to avoid conversation. Leo was more than happy for me to go to Wisconsin alone, and I was happy to leave him in Las Vegas.

The whole point in going home is to visit with family, including aunts, uncles, and cousins. You go to someone's house and you sit around and visit, which involves talking. Ben was a good talker, and perhaps it was his amicability that resulted in my mom inviting him to take part in our family photo session at my brother Tony's farm, which was where my mom grew up. I had no plans to invite him to join us and expected him to wait patiently inside Tony's century-old, heated farmhouse while the rest of us froze outside in Wisconsin's December cold, posing in front of the barn, for the sake of a few photos.

It had been years since we'd had family photos taken; there was no need for a man I'd been dating for five months to be in them. But for some reason, Mom invited Ben to be part of it, and for some reason, he accepted. As we walked toward the barn, I thought, Ben and I can position ourselves on the end of the group so that, if we broke up (God forbid!), I can photoshop him out of the picture. However, the photographer decided Ben and I needed to be in the center of the group! I could've opened my mouth to say what I was thinking, that it was too early for Ben to be part of our family photos, but it felt too awkward, so we moved to the center.

I also could've protested that it was too soon for us to travel halfway across the country and stay with my family. Even though my fear of being single with herpes would ensure my relationship with Ben lasted my lifetime, I still had my doubts. I didn't mind not meeting his parents so soon into our relationship, and he should have given me the same consideration when it came to my family. However, Ben's ex-wife had cheated on him while she was traveling, and her infidelity led to him believing that it was inappropriate for a person in a relationship to travel alone.

The cheating had started after his ex attended her twenty-year high school reunion and became reacquainted with old friends. That reacquaintance turned into regular gatherings for drinks, to which Ben was not invited because Deborah said he didn't know her friends and he wouldn't feel comfortable around them. That was her cover story. But in reality, she needed to go out alone in order to cultivate a relationship with an old high school flame, Wrench Boy.

Her cheating was why he insisted on coming home with me for Christmas so soon after we'd started dating. I didn't push back because

I understood his reasoning and I wanted him to know that he could trust me. But I also worried that he'd find Wisconsin boring.

Traveling to meet my family would have been a different story if they'd lived in Las Vegas or somewhere that was within driving distance; Ben would've had an escape if the visit didn't go well. But there was no escape in Wisconsin, and he'd have to stick it out once he saw for himself the lack of amenities in my hometown and the amount of sitting around required in visiting family. The guy liked to move around and keep busy, and I worried that he, like Leo, would find Wisconsin not to his liking and ruin my trip home.

Wisconsin wasn't our first excursion together. The two of us had already visited Puerto Vallarta, Mexico, a couple months earlier in October. It was a test, Ben said, to see how we would travel together. As he explained, we already knew we were sexually compatible, and we enjoyed each other's company. Since seeing the world was important to him, we needed to know how we would do in that arena. Once we established that we were compatible as traveling companions, the forward momentum of our relationship would be sealed.

Unlike the other girlfriends Ben had prior to my arrival, I'd paid for my part of the Mexico trip and we'd pooled our cash to jointly pay for meals and any other expenses. I wanted him to see that I could pull my own weight financially, not just in terms of paying my bills, but in being responsible with my money. I was showing him that I could afford a trip from time to time without going into debt or mooching off his success. Ben said I was the first girlfriend he'd had post-divorce who could afford to travel, and he liked that. The trip to Mexico had been a victory.

On the flight home from Wisconsin after the Christmas trip, I thanked Ben for being him and mixing so well with my family. I meant it. Despite the braggadocious things he'd said here and there to my relatives that made me cringe, his ability to blend with my family helped me make the decision to move into his house.

I wanted to start *really* blending with his family. And the way to blend, Ben and I both agreed, was to move in and be around all the time, rather than just make appearances at dinners and at the kids' extracurricular activities. And besides, I told myself continually, my house was still there; I would just rent it, not sell it.

The plan was for me to move in with my two cats during his non-custodial week, without giving the kids a heads-up that I'd be there the next time they came around. He thought Eli and Maddie would have an easier time accepting my intrusion into their home if they didn't have any other choice but to accept that I was already there. Plus, Eli believed he was allergic to "some cats," but not all cats. To persuade him that he'd be ok with my cats, Ben thought it would be better to not tell Eli the cats were in the house. When he had no reaction, it would prove that he wasn't allergic to them.

Eli and Maddie seemed to like being sick or injured. Eli continually complained of allergies and stomach illnesses, while Maddie often wore braces on her wrists and knees for supposed injuries to her muscles and joints. They were weak, attention-seeking kids with weird and—I believed—nonexistent pains and illnesses.

Ben's kids and my two nieces back in Wisconsin, who were about the same age as Ben's sons, were as different as night and day. Rachel and Rilee were strong girls who hunted with my sister and her husband. They weren't coddled. They were nice and had good social skills around adults. They worked jobs rather than waiting for handouts from their parents. Rachel had documented allergies and irritable bowel syndrome that didn't keep her down, whereas Eli went to doctors and medical specialists only to be told repeatedly that there was nothing wrong with him physically. Still, his parents indulged his need to be sick and allergic and scheduled his medical appointments. I wondered why they couldn't just tell him to knock it off.

Eli was at his father's house for a full twenty-four hours before he realized there had been cats cohabiting in the house with him the entire time. Since my cats were new to the house and the people in it, they spent most of their first couple weeks hiding under Ben's bed. But they had been stealthily checking out every corner of the house prior to the kids' arrival, and there's no way, if Eli were truly allergic to cats, that he wouldn't have been affected by their dander. As I suspected, he was not.

About my presence in the house, Eli asked Ben as they passed each other on the stairs to the second floor, "Does she live here now?"

Ben said his reply to Eli was a simple *yes* and the conversation ended. Ben continued down the stairs and Eli continued up. The girl, he said, spoke not a word about my presence.

Maybe the kids were so used to Ben's girlfriends moving in that they didn't have much to say about their new roommate. Or maybe Ben was lying and the kids had lots to say about yet another woman moving into their living space. If they did, Ben didn't tell me. Or maybe Eli and Maddie discussed in private, to each other, how they were going to be noncomplying assholes to me. But it didn't matter—I wasn't looking for a best friend in any of Ben's kids; my hope was that we'd develop a routine that involved respect and acceptance of each other over time, and I waited hopefully for that to happen.

I didn't bring a lot of my worldly possessions to Ben's house because his was mostly furnished. I showed up with a few wooden pieces that were either gifts or in good shape, such as a bookcase given to me by my mom, as well as a dresser, two end tables, a TV stand, and a coffee table. The bookcase and my other pieces matched and came from the same store that sold pine furniture made in Mexico. None of it was expensive, but I liked the rustic look of it and it fit with my farmhouse style, which was nowhere near Ben's modern style. My stuff didn't complement the black furniture in Ben's house, but I liked it and I wanted to bring it with me.

Ben's plan was for me to hurry up and rent my house while I lived with him. With his guidance and pressure, I started the process. My house needed to be empty for the incoming tenants, so I had to get rid of most of the stuff I'd accumulated over the past eleven years.

I hired a junk hauler to remove a few large items and put the rest of what I didn't want out in a garage sale one Saturday. As it turned out, very few of my items were sellable, so I ended up putting it all in the garage.

I took a whole three months to clean and gut my home of everything in it. Ben wanted the rental income to start flowing as soon as possible. My mortgage was $600 per month, and I could get $1200 monthly through rent. I had agreed to pay Ben $400 each month to reside in his house, so my net earnings on the rent would be $200. I didn't mind paying Ben rent in the least; this was yet another way to show him I wasn't a mooch.

Renting my house scared me. It was my safety net and I was afraid to lose it in case living with Ben didn't go well. But I was also scared renters would destroy my place. I'd heard horror stories of the damage renters had done to properties and worried about the expense of paying for fixes if that happened with my tenants.

Ben had owned rental properties in the past. He had had to sell a fourplex he and his wife owned together as part of their divorce settlement. He wasn't afraid of tenants with bad credit, of which there are many in Las Vegas. His philosophy was that if they came to view the rental with enough cash for the security deposit and first month's rent, and they had proof of employment with paystubs that showed they made enough to cover their monthly rent, then sign the lease on the spot. And that's the advice I took when I was eventually ready to let my safety net go.

Ben was with me when a short, blonde girl in her twenties, as wide as she was tall, came to see the house. She brought her cosigner, her heavyset Filipino boyfriend, as well as her large mom and normal-sized dad, with her to view the house. The dad was Black and obviously not her biological father, but she introduced him as if he was. All four seemed like nice people. The young couple had the cash for the security deposit and first month's rent, they proved they were properly employed, and they were ready to sign the lease.

I still hadn't cleaned out the garage and asked the new renters if they were interested in any of the items. All the Christmas decorations I'd been given over the years were in there; I couldn't take them to a Jewish home. Even though Christmas was just a holiday to me and I didn't celebrate the religious origins of the day, I knew Ben would have no part in decorations that signified the great divide between the Jews and Christians. I had no problem leaving those things behind and took only my snowmen, which signified nothing more than the happy and fun side of winter.

A large wooden dresser and some kitchens items were also in the garage; there just wasn't room for those things in Ben's house and I had to let them go. Ben's house was stocked with more than enough kitchen supplies from his Israeli girlfriend. The blonde and her boyfriend said to leave the items, and they'd take what they wanted and toss the rest. That solved my problem.

Toward the end of my tenant's one-year lease, I received a notice from code enforcement that my tenants had violated the city's garage sale ordinance by holding more than the allotted two garage sales per month. It wasn't until after I evicted them for non-payment of rent that I found out from my neighbors the true nuisance my renters had created for the neighborhood. A strange lady came every weekend and held sales from my garage with my stuff and, presumably, other items she and my renters accumulated to sell in their joint thrift business. I guess if I'd had their tenacity, I might've been able to offload more of my stuff rather than providing things for my tenants to try and sell weekend after weekend.

Chapter 13

Life In My New Home

S oon after I moved in, Ben and I started an online business together selling meal replacement bars and hygiene products from a multi-level marketing company, except we weren't part of the pyramid of sellers around the world selling the products on the up-and-up. Ben had a friend in Israel who was high on the pyramid and had no interest in selling the products. He was making enough money from the people underneath him that the effort to sell shampoo and granola bars was beneath him. However, he had to purchase a certain amount of product to maintain his placement in the marketing scheme. That friend shipped the products to Ben to do with them as Ben pleased, which was to have me sell the stuff on eBay.

Our plan was to use any money we made from our sales to sponsor our entertainment expenses, such as eating out and movies. It sounded fine to me—Ben was very generous with his money and paid the majority of our expenses, and he did so without complaint, without even a hint that I needed to contribute a cent toward our fun. I was more than happy to contribute to our partnership and pull my financial weight by using my spare time to package and ship our sales.

When Ben said his name couldn't be associated with our online store because he worried about the effect it could have on his contractor and business licenses, I willingly put our store, along with the associated PayPal account, in my name only.

I found it fun posting items for sale on eBay and watching the sales come in. I boxed up the orders in the evening and dropped them off at the post office on my way to work the following morning. It was a nice little system going that required no overhead except the purchase of boxes, packing supplies, and postage.

Our profits went straight to a debit card that I'd connected to our store; as planned, we used what we made on entertainment expenses. When it came time to pay for meals at restaurants, I whipped out the card.

I had no idea what Ben feared would happen with our store until the eBay account I created eventually received a cease-and-desist letter from a law firm. The letter said that I wasn't allowed to sell the products and that the firm would pursue legal action against me if I didn't stop. I hadn't known I was doing anything wrong by reselling products that had been legitimately purchased by someone who had the right to do so. Ben most certainly did, though, and was willing to take the risk as long as his name wasn't tied to the venture.

I thought it was pretty crappy of Ben to expose me to potential legal trouble by selling those products. It hurt my heart a little to know he would've let me take the fall for a few bucks. Once I received the order to stop selling, I shut down our store and the business was over. Ben wanted me to sell the remaining items we had in stock before shutting down but I refused. The remaining hair products and meal replacement bars took up space in his house for a long time afterward. Our online business lasted about six months.

· · · · ●· · ● · · · ·

In those days, I was driving a new, boxy, compact Kia Soul that I loved. However, Ben said I needed a bigger car to accommodate his family when Tyler was also around. The huge pickup truck Ben used for work had an extended cab that could fit Ben and me and all three of his kids easily. Every two years he traded in his vehicle for a tax write-off and therefore always drove the newest of the new pickups available on the market. A larger SUV for me, he said, would be easier for all of us to get in and out of, more economical on gas, and provide more maneuverability on city streets and in parking garages and lots. Since our goal was to eventually get married, why wait, he asked, to get a car that suited our needs as a family?

I rolled with his logic and willingly traded in my small Kia for the larger Kia Sportage. Ben did all the negotiating with the salesman at the dealership and it was wonderful—I was happy and relaxed with Ben doing all the talking. His steamroller approach to negotiation angered the salesman at times, but I walked away with a car at close to the same payment I'd had with my Soul. It was refreshing to think I'd never have to negotiate with any salespeople or home repair people ever again.

I'd been willing to make a trade for a car that Ben felt better suited his family as long as it met my criteria: I wanted loan payments low enough so that I could easily pay it off well in advance of the end of the loan, and it needed to have enough storage space to carry my craft sale supplies.

Making and selling crafts was my hobby. I painted gourds, turning them into cute holiday subjects, such as witches, snowmen, and Santa Clauses. My specialty was Christmas tree ornaments—they sold like hotcakes at craft sales. My parents grew and dried my gourds for me in the Wisconsin countryside, which helped to keep my supply costs down. It also created a good, wholesome story that the ladies who bought my wares seemed to like.

I'd taken up decorative painting not long after Leo and I moved to the San Francisco Bay area at the start of our marriage. We were new to California and knew no one; I was bored and needed a pastime. I'd always been fond of folk-art painting—doll faces, flowers, country scenes, cute signs, etc. To my delight, I found a craft shop nearby that offered decorative painting classes and I signed up. I had artistic ability and I picked up the folk-art painting technique easily.

To learn to paint, we usually used a wooden surface of some sort—a box, a picture frame, flat pieces of wood. We learned on other surfaces as well, including glass jars and metal. In one of my classes, we converted a birdhouse gourd into a snowman with a painted winter scene around the bottom half. From that point forward, I was hooked on gourds. I liked that they were natural products that had once been seeds and, after drying out, became rock-hard, perfect painting surfaces.

Eventually I had boxes full of gourds in my North Las Vegas garage—more than I could ever paint. My mom would ship them to me or throw them in the back of her minivan and drive them out to me if she was visiting. She was a great gourd pusher!

My boxes of unpainted gourds ended up in Ben's garage after I moved in. He was nice enough to buy shelves so that I could organize and stack my stash efficiently and out of the way. However, he was not so congenial when it came to the commitment I made to my hobby.

Getting ready for craft sales required painting tons of gourds, which was very time-consuming and a solo project. He said that rather than being alone with my craft, I could be in the living room watching TV with him and his kids.

Leo didn't mind me painting the gourds. I'd set up a small desk in our dining room, which was connected to our living room, so that I could see and hear the TV as I painted. He was often lounging on the living room couch watching TV or reclined with his laptop open. He'd position the screen in such a way that I wouldn't be able to see what he was looking at if I were to suddenly get up and head his way. Whatever the case, my ability to keep myself occupied was Leo's asset. To Ben, it was senseless that I'd rather paint alone than hang out with him and his family.

Part of the issue was that my painting area in Ben's house was way out of the way, upstairs in our bedroom, so I was separated from everyone. We could've set it up for me in a common area; however, Ben wanted the clutter of my painting supplies hidden away. So, I brought the small, cheap pressboard desk I'd used at my house, along with my paints, brushes, and other supplies, and together, Ben and I set me up in a corner of our bedroom, next to his much larger, custom-made office desk where he wrote up estimates for clients and did accounting work for his business. Admittedly, I was fine being isolated because I wasn't quite comfortable with his kids and liked having a place to hide.

Ben was impressed with my painting abilities and wanted me to decorate the house with gourds I'd painted. He even tried to pawn off one of my ghosts on Maddie, who was a fan of the *Nightmare Before Christmas* movie. She replied that the gourd was "creepy" and that she didn't want it. It was fine by me that she had no care for my gourd. It was also fine by me not to decorate the house with any of my work. Cute gourds didn't match the esthetic of this modern house with Jewish symbolism all over the place.

Ben appreciated my talent, but he wasn't quite on board with me trying to make a business out of it. Soon after I moved in, I was hired by a garden store in Wisconsin to paint Halloween-themed gourds. It took a lot of time to finish those gourds by the store's deadline, which was time away from him and the kids.

Ben said the return on my investment was too low and he couldn't understand why I spent so much time on something that didn't produce a lot of cash. Finding a product to sell, like the supplements and hygiene products we sold illegally, was a better option, he said, because it required less time investment and the profit margin was greater. I told him painting was my talent and I enjoyed doing it. Even the smallest profit was acceptable to me.

Painting was just my hobby; my real dream was to be a writer. Using crafting and painting as a creative outlet satisfied me until the day when I'd finally put on paper all the ideas floating around in my head. I was going to get at it someday, but until then, I would paint and sell my gourds, which fit nicely, when boxed up for transport to sales, in my square Kia Soul, and later my Kia Sportage.

• • • • ● • ● • • • •

Soon after I started tooling around in my Sportage, we loaded up my car and headed for the port of San Diego—Ben, the kids, and I were going on a cruise. Maddie and Eli had been on a trip with their mom a week or two earlier and I soon noticed a pattern developing. If the mother scheduled a trip with the kids, Ben almost immediately planned a getaway to a California amusement park or somewhere else that required an overnight stay. Ben denied that he was in a competition with Deborah to show the kids a better time, but the timing all but screamed of a rivalry. Still, this cruise to Mexico would be my first vacation with Ben's children and I hoped I'd have a bit of a breakthrough, returning to Las Vegas as their friend.

Ben was in the driver's seat, I was in the passenger seat, and the kids were in the back. My traveling companions had been on several cruises in the past, some of them extravagant by Ben's telling, and most of them paid for by his ex-wife's wealthy father. This would be my first and I was excited, even though I was still invisible to at least one person in the car.

Eli and I had developed somewhat of a friendship; of the three kids, he was my favorite. But there was one issue: he made eating out anywhere a real test in patience for all involved. After our meals came to a close, he would pick up his phone and head to the restroom, where he'd spend fifteen minutes to half an hour attempting to poop. He said the urge to defecate was there, along with stomach discomfort, and he had to wait it out perched on a toilet to see if his bowels would make a move. All the while the rest of us sat at our table, bill paid, and waited. Still, he was a far better travel companion—at least in terms of friendliness toward me—than his little sister.

Ben's friend, David, was the one who'd come up with the idea for the cruise—he'd found a killer deal, booked the trip for his family, and told Ben about it. David somehow finagled incredible deals on whatever he was in the market to purchase, whether it was a trip, a business, or a home. As he told it, in the negotiations for these deals, the selling side was always clamoring—for some ungodly reason—to provide him with the lowest price, with the most amenities, possible. When he and Shuli sold their house and purchased a new one in a gated community, David said the seller liked him so much that he lowered the price by thousands of dollars to ensure David's family would follow through on buying it.

So much bullshit came out of that man's mouth.

His wife was just as bad, except instead of people liking her so much that they threw deals at her, she bragged of using her wits and sharp tongue to get bargains. Every day, she said, she traveled to six Ross stores, keeping her eyes on the already reduced-priced items she wanted until they were reduced even more.

Six stores...

Every day...

There was no item of clothing or knickknack in this world that would've gotten me to put that much effort into shopping for it.

When Shuli invited me to go with her to a craft class at a Michael's hobby store, Ben encouraged me to go, hoping that she and I would bond over our interest in crafting. What a great convenience it would've been for him to have his lady become friends with his best friend's wife.

The project we signed up for involved painting with acrylic paints. I'd brought my supply of paintbrushes that I'd accumulated over the years, which I stored in a handmade and well-worn travel pouch that I bought when I first started taking painting classes in my twenties. I didn't have the most expensive brushes, but I had many different kinds and I treated them well to make sure they'd last year after year. Shuli brought a supply of makeup brushes she had on hand. I soon learned she wasn't being a friend to the environment by repurposing those makeup tools into painting brushes; she was being downright, 100 percent cheap.

When we arrived at the class, we were told by the teacher that we'd need to go into the store to buy a small bottle of acrylic paint to complete our projects. At the cash register, Shuli, who supposedly had a few million dollars in the bank, rudely demanded the cashier give her a discount—on a $1.25 bottle of paint! I can't remember the reason why she demanded the discount, but I do recall the disgust I felt at her level of cheapness. The woman at the register had a 40 percent-off coupon from that week's sales paper and allowed Shuli to use it. I had no problem paying full price for my paint.

That craft class was the first and last one I took with Shuli. If I had to deal with her at her Shabbat and holiday dinners to honor my commitment to Ben, I sure wasn't going to spend my free time with her as well.

David and Shuli's frequent Shabbat and holiday dinners often included another Israeli couple or two; Shuli seemed to have a knack for finding Israeli couples to invite. Once she overheard a man talking in Hebrew on his cell phone while in the checkout line at a grocery store, and he and his wife ended up at Shuli's dining room table. It was as if they were attempting to create a strong network of friends to replace the extended family they didn't have because Shuli's family was in Israel and David was estranged from his. The only problem was that the friendships didn't stick.

At these dinner parties, I'd usually end up sitting near the kids' table and talking to the children in English while the adults spoke in Hebrew. The conversation amongst the adults would start in English, no doubt for my benefit, but would slowly change over to the others' native tongue. It didn't bother me too much—I'd shift my attention over to the kids to see what kind of conversation I could get out of them, or I'd turn to my phone for entertainment while the people around me talked and laughed.

After sitting through a dinner or two, the newfound friends would never be seen again. According to Shuli, the excuse most gave for not returning to her parties was that they were headed out of town or had a mysterious "other" commitment. I asked Ben if he noticed the pattern that the couples and their kids would drop out of sight after only one or two dinners. To me it seemed obvious that David and Shuli were intolerable fools that smart people avoided. Why, I asked, were we the only constant presence in their home? Ben had no explanation other than that he liked talking to David and enjoyed Shuli's cooking.

Due to Ben's weird friendship with David, and that we'd planned our cruise on David's recommendation, I expected that our two groups would spend all our time together, both on the ship and on landside excursions. I wondered how it would work considering Maddie ignored Maserati, and there were at least ten years in age difference between Eli and their son, Lee. But I told myself repeatedly that at least I was going to sunny Mexico, and that would be enough to make our travel companions tolerable. However, it became apparent quickly after boarding the ship that Ben would make no effort to coordinate plans with the other family while cruising. Our time together was limited to running into each other in the dining area.

Ben said David asked him why our groups seemed to always be on different schedules and at different locations. Ben's reply was that he didn't want to revolve our plans around six-year-old Lee. Ben said he knew what it was like to travel with small children because he'd done it with his own. He didn't want our cruise experience to be dictated by when the little boy ate, napped, and played. I had no problem with that very true excuse!

The cruise with Ben, Maddie, and Eli was actually enjoyable. The four of us hung out together, and even though Maddie mostly ignored me, certain moments with her were promising. At those times, I could feel an air of hope that, with time and patience, we could develop a friendship. One of those moments turned out to be a treasure hunt of sorts in search of a gross Mexican lollipop covered in red chili powder.

It turned out that Maddie loved those suckers, so on an excursion into Acapulco, Mexico, I used the Spanish I'd learned in college, living in Mexico, and from my Mexican ex-husband, to search for them in a grocery store and a couple small corner stores. I knew the suckers she wanted and had tried them once upon a time. The chili powder on the outside of the candy could make your lips pucker and your eyes roll back in your head. No way I would've gone searching for them unless a little girl who hated me liked them and I could earn some points by helping her locate one.

She and I entered the stores together while Ben and Eli waited outside. I got a slight feeling that she thought I was cool because I could speak to Mexicans in their language to ask about those suckers, which we found at the third store.

Early on in our cruise, she asked me, while lounging in our cramped cabin before heading to the all-you-could-eat breakfast buffet, if I knew how to French braid hair.

"Dawn, do you know how to French braid hair?" She actually looked at me and asked her question directly to me, not through her father or brother.

I told her the truth; I used to have long hair that I French braided, but it was more than twenty years in the past and I wasn't sure if I still had the ability. With that answer, she turned away from me and said not a word to me the rest of the cruise. Ben asked me on Maddie's behalf to help her find the lollipop.

Not long after that cruise, on yet another trip to Wisconsin, I discovered that I still could braid. I twisted both my teenage nieces' long hair into multiple braids—two on one girl's head and four on the other. It became a tradition after this initial braiding that, every time I visited Wisconsin, I'd weave their hair into as many French braids as each girl desired.

I loved the fact that my nieces wanted me to braid their hair. When they learned I'd be staying with them in their homes for a visit, they'd say I couldn't return to Las Vegas until their hair was braided. It was fun bonding time spent with my sister's daughters.

I sometimes wondered after the cruise what would have happened if I'd braided Maddie's hair. Rather than say I wasn't sure I remembered how to do it, I should've told her it had been a long time since I'd attempted a braid, but that I'd be more than happy to give it a shot with her hair. Given that my ability came back fairly easily with my nieces, Maddie's braids would have turned out beautiful. Perhaps we would've bonded over the experience and repeated it back home in her father's house in Las Vegas. Maybe we would have become friends.

Chapter 14
The Fuck Fest

Ben and I stood outside the locked and secured front door of Desert Mountain Institute just outside of Palm Springs, California. He spoke to a woman through an intercom, telling her that we had a reservation for two. He'd called earlier from our hotel to book our stay, which they'd held with a credit card. She checked her records, saw that we were on the list, and said she'd come to let us in.

Desert Mountain Institute advertised itself online as a clothing-optional resort and day spa when it was, in fact, a swingers' club. The "spa" disguised itself so well online that on Ben's first visit, he hadn't realized until after arriving with his Deborah that it was a downright fuck fest. This is how I came to refer to Desert Mountain after seeing the activities that went on inside that place. It was a fuck fest.

Ben said that, as he and Deborah started to experience marital difficulties, he'd suggested they attend Desert Mountain to spice up their love life. Deborah apparently showed no apprehension or desire to flee after learning the true nature of the place upon their arrival. According to Ben, she'd engaged in girl-on-girl activity not long after entering the club, which he thoroughly enjoyed watching.

Despite the girl-on-girl activity, he and Deborah did not swap partners with other couples. They had the opportunity on at least one occasion, but Deborah wouldn't agree to have sex with the husband, so Ben couldn't have sex with the wife. But she apparently enjoyed Desert Mountain enough that she agreed to multiple subsequent visits.

Deborah went on to become friends with several women at the resort. When they planned return visits, she texted the "friends" she'd made to coordinate trips at the same time. The way it sounded to me, Deborah tried to normalize their visits to Palm Springs by making it appear as if they weren't going to a swingers' club; they were going to hang out with friends. They'd sit naked in the hot tub with these friends and catch up on their goings-on since they'd last seen each other; they'd lie naked in the sun together on lounge chairs strewn about the compound; they'd leave to have dinner together and then return to the club for more friendly bonding.

I had no desire to form friendships with anybody there and I didn't.

The resort sat on a residential street where it had no business existing. I could imagine such a place in the middle of the desert with no neighbors around, but this establishment was on a dead-end road lined with about ten to fifteen houses directly across from it. The houses looked fairly new, at least no more than twenty years old, and middle-class, the type of dwellings you'd expect new families to be able to afford. When Leo and I bought our house in North Las Vegas, we had to sign a disclosure saying that we knew the house was located near a pig farm and that we might smell pig manure from time to time. I wondered what kind of disclosure each of these homeowners had to sign.

Ben said one of the houses toward the end of the street belonged to a husband and wife who were Desert Mountain regulars. He'd gotten to know the couple, who were in their seventies, during his many visits with his ex-wife and with at least one of the girlfriends who came before me. The couple told Ben they enjoyed this swingers' club so much that they'd bought the house for easy access to the fuck fest. They usually visited Desert Mountain with two other elderly couples whose company they apparently enjoyed very much, which I witnessed for myself as they swapped partners within their group and screwed in the open.

The land on either side of Desert Mountain was vacant. It seemed weird that an investor hadn't built a commercial structure or more homes on that open land. The club hadn't stopped people from occupying the houses on the other side of the street, so it seemed logical that they'd live next to it as well. I wondered what came first—the housing or the swingers' club. Desert Mountain's building looked older than the neighboring residences and was probably some sort of hotel/spa before it was sold and converted into a swingers' club. How it had been allowed to exist in a residential area seemed odd, as if shenanigans and illegal payments must have exchanged hands for it to open doors in the first place, as well as to continue to operate.

The lack of development around Desert Mountain was actually good for the sex club, not because there were fewer prying eyes to worry about, but because the vacant land made a perfect parking lot for patrons. There were about twenty to thirty cars parked in the dirt around the facility, including the convertible sports car Ben had wanted to purchase jointly with me.

I felt like a complete pervert standing outside this place waiting to be let in. Desert Mountain was hardly a good neighbor, with club music blaring from behind the ten-foot walls surrounding it. Desert Mountain seemed to be taunting the neighbors with noise, as if to say that everybody knew what was going on and there was nothing any of them could do about it.

After the longest twenty-minute wait of my life, a topless brunette in her thirties greeted us with the office phone in hand. It was cordless and old-fashioned, but I suppose it worked just as well as a more modern earpiece would have, so that she wouldn't miss a call while ushering us into the building. She wore a maxi skirt from the waist down.

Upon passing the threshold, I immediately spied naked bodies everywhere. There was no safe place for my eyes to look. Naked people were scattered in all directions, hanging out in and alongside the pool, lounging on patio chairs, and walking about here and there. Some were having sex. As we were escorted by the topless lady to the office to pay our $200 entrance fee, I could only gaze up at the sky or look down at my feet to avoid taking in the nudity and sexual activity.

Desert Mountain Institute wasn't about being comfortable in your own naked skin and admiring the human form. It was about fucking your wife or girlfriend in public with people watching and then fucking another man's wife while you watched her husband fucking your woman. I'd even heard of men indulging in other men while their wives were off indulging in other men, too.

The people at this fuck fest wanted to be seen. It was unbelievable to me the things they were doing out in the open. Ben obliged by staring intently at everyone leisurely lying about and actively fucking, while I took quick peeks.

Inside the office, Ben handed over $200 in cash to the topless lady and made sure there would be no charge to the credit card number he provided over the phone to hold our reservation. He typically used his credit card for all purchases so that he'd have a record of the transaction for a potential tax write-off, but this expenditure, he wanted no record of.

In exchange for our payment, the topless lady attached a white, plastic band to each of our left wrists. This band was our ticket to come in and out of the Institute for the rest of the day and night.

She also gave us two thin, red, ratty towels that felt and looked as if they'd been used by countless naked people before us and washed hundreds of times. There must have been at least seventy-five people patronizing this place while we were there. With all of them paying $200 per couple, or much more if they were staying in the hotel rooms inside the compound, you would've thought the Desert Mountain could've sprung for new towels from Walmart every now and again. Or maybe since the place's true intent was to allow people to be at their dirtiest and most perverted, there was no need for niceties like fluffy towels.

I generally liked to chip in on the cost of our excursions, or at least offer to do so, but when it came time to pay the topless lady, I made no effort to reach for my wallet. This trip, which included a four-hour drive to get here, was purely to satisfy his sexual need and he could pay for it.

It would never have occurred to me to go to a swingers' club if it weren't for Ben steamrolling me into coming. He said this fuck fest relaxed him, and I felt like if I didn't at least visit this place once, it would become a source of contention between us, possibly leading to a breakup. My fear of being single with herpes was greater than my fear of whatever happened at a fuck fest.

Not soon after starting the drive to Palm Springs and before we'd even left Las Vegas' jurisdiction, Ben had tried to calm my nerves by offering me the same agreement he'd had with Deborah—we wouldn't participate in any swinging unless we both agreed upon it. His words of assurance only made my stomach turn with nausea and increase my level of fear that he did indeed want to swap with other couples. Upon agreeing to give the Institute a shot at least once, I told Ben that I would not engage in any swinging, yet here he was speaking as if it might still be an option. I feared that, if he found someone he wanted to screw, he'd push me to participate.

Up until this point, only Jerry knew that I had herpes and I had no idea who Ben told. Ben and I couldn't have sex with people at the Institute without disclosing ourselves as carriers; it would have been unethical not to do so. Was that his plan—to tell people? No way was I going to admit my status to strangers and potentially face rejection by people who would have sex with anybody but me.

The topless lady asked us if we'd each like a margarita. Ben declined and I accepted the offer. I'd already had a can of malt liquor from a gas station we stopped at during the short drive from the hotel; I hoped to relieve some of the fear and nausea I felt about coming to a place like this. Even though I had a couple more cans of liquid courage in a plastic shopping bag, I wasn't going to turn down a free drink—I needed all the help I could get.

With our towels in hand, we followed the staffer to a little kitchenette, which was stocked with soft drinks and bottled water in a refrigerator. There was also a selection of chips, crackers, and cookies, and a rotating hot dog warmer, like the ones you'd see at a gas station convenience store. All these snacks and beverages were available for the taking by naked patrons. It was weird—and a bit funny—to me that chips and hot dogs were there for patrons to indulge in between fucks.

The topless lady pulled out margarita mix and tequila from another fridge, which also housed bottles of wine, and poured me a drink. She asked if we needed a tour of the facility; we declined, as Ben knew the place well. He said he'd show me to the lockers where we were to take off all our clothes and stash our valuables. Nudity was mandatory.

Ben knew the drill and his clothes came off easily. I followed suit, removing my clothes and placing them in our locker. I'd brought the lock and key I used at my Pilates studio; normally I'd put the key in my yoga pants pocket while I worked out, but since I was in the buff, I hung the key from the wristband provided by the staff. I prayed I didn't lose the key, as I didn't want to return to our hotel naked!

The Institute had rooms to rent, which would've made things easier for us. However, Ben said the cost of renting a room, even though it included the entrance fee, was too much. He'd learned through his many trips there with his wife that it was cheaper to rent a hotel room down the road for a hundred bucks a night and pay the daily rate. The wristbands would allow us to leave, go eat something more substantial than chips, and come back.

To get an idea of how Desert Mountain was laid out, think of a self-contained Mexican hacienda with tall walls around the perimeter and a large open-air courtyard in the middle. In the olden days, you would've found a protected community of people and animals residing inside the four walls, with living quarters and sheds or barns. The stucco walls and tiled roof were also in the hacienda style, which fit in with the surrounding desert area quite nicely, unless, of course, you knew what was going on inside that one-story building.

Once inside, I could see that the courtyard was the heart of the complex. People were in the pool, the oversized hot tub, or lying on lounge chairs. A party room with disco lights and dance floor separated the pool from the hot tub. After the sun went down, the guests would dance in there to music provided by a DJ, or they would screw on the large, round, red velvet bed placed conveniently at the edge of the dance floor.

Despite the club's Mexican architectural style, Desert Mountain was decorated with Buddha statues and Buddhist symbolism from wall to wall. I didn't get the connection between Buddhism and a fuck fest until, approximately a year later, I learned that Buddha was a cover after the club's owner, Georgi, opened a similar "Buddhist worship center" in a residential area in Las Vegas. He disguised his fuck fests as places of worship to trick zoning and building departments into approving his supposed religious sanctuaries. Somehow that story worked in Palm Springs, but not in Las Vegas. Clark County, which had jurisdiction over the Nevada facility, eventually listened to complaining neighbors and shut down the bogus temple of love despite the many Buddha statues.

Georgi had talked to Ben about providing remodeling services for his Las Vegas expansion; however, he ultimately went with another contractor because Ben was not about to violate building codes or break any other law to make the Las Vegas temple happen. As much as Ben loved the Palm Springs place, he said he'd never be a patron to a fuck fest in our backyard for fear he'd be seen by someone he knew.

Inside Desert Mountain in Palm Springs, it was downright weird walking around naked. Ben wanted to sit in the hot tub, but I wasn't ready to be close to other naked people yet. He walked me over to the sunbathing section, where we spread our cheap towels on two chairs side by side and lay down. Many empty chairs had red towels on them, which held the chairs for their temporary owners who were off enjoying the club's amenities.

I had the same impression of the chairs as I did the towels. Upon walking into this place, you couldn't tell with a quick glance its age and maintenance needs. But now sitting and observing and looking closely at my surroundings, I saw neglect in the chairs and in a nearby tiki barbeque and bar area that was unmanned by a bartender or cook. People were sitting on the barstools with their own drinks and food, which they had delivered or brought in themselves from local eateries. The aged and weathered look of everything made me wonder at the financial viability of the place.

After several minutes, Ben couldn't stand being sedentary any longer and headed toward the hot tub. He was an antsy guy and needed movement. After about thirty minutes of soaking in the sun and attempting to read an e-book on my phone, I felt comfortable enough to join him in the spa.

Walking around naked was weird, at least at first. I got used to it quickly though, finding it easier to be naked than in a bikini. I tried to find swimsuits that covered as much cellulite as possible, which usually ended up being a pair of swim shorts. Being naked was different. With swim shorts or a one-piece, you can hide cellulite or a pouchy belly. But nudity provides no safety, a fact that hit me soon after entering Desert Mountain and seeing all types of naked bodies that were far from hard, muscular, or toned. Nobody was hiding any imperfections at this place, and it made me feel comfortable.

Most of the people were middle-aged or older. I saw lots of stretch marks on women's midriffs and was a little weirded out thinking these women had kids waiting for them back home. Sometimes you could see apprehension from the women, similar to my misgivings, and you knew they were there to satisfy some weird curiosity in their husbands. Others seemed to be having the time of their lives.

Ben was pleasantly surprised to see me join him in the hot tub so soon after our arrival. He compared me to his Israeli girlfriend who needed much more time to feel comfortable enough to join him in the bubbling water. He told me I was doing better than her on her first—and only—trip to the fuck fest. She demanded they leave after less than a couple hours. I had to make my stay last longer than hers, and I did. We stayed in that hot tub from mid-afternoon until early evening.

In the hot tub we talked to several couples and watched the go-ings-on around us. Some conversations were completely normal even though we were naked and people would often be having sex within our sights. Many of the couples were from Southern California, while a good number were from places all over the country. We discussed our cities of residence, our occupations, and where Ben was from. His accent and whiteness threw people off; most thought he was European and were pleasantly surprised to find out he was Israeli.

Even though Desert Mountain didn't advertise itself as a fuck fest on its website, word got around. From these people in the hot tub, I learned that there were cruises, clubs, and hotel conventions across the country specifically for swingers. Once you went to one event, you found out through word of mouth about others.

Most of our conversations were tame and I'm sure couples could tell that we weren't there to swing, or "play," as they said, after very little chatter. Some would ask outright if we were there to observe or play. Ben always said to observe, which made me happy and eased my mind.

As time went on and the sun went down, people shifted from the pool to the spa. Where the pool had once been the gathering spot, now the hot tub became the place to be. Toward the end of our evening at Desert Mountain, a forty-ish lady named Susan moved over next to us and struck up a conversation. She was White, attractive and with a medium build—neither fat nor skinny. She didn't ask us outright if we were there to play, but she was probably trying to feel us out.

We talked to Susan for quite a while about business and her property investments near the beach in Southern California, and she gave us background information on Desert Mountain. She said she was good friends with Georgi, and that the city council had no problem with this club existing in a residential area; in fact, they welcomed it. She talked about the purifying water in the pool and spa, claiming that it came from underground thermal sources and had healing properties.

I didn't believe most of what she said, but the conversation was at least interesting.

Then another woman entered the hot tub, and I noticed Susan's eyes lock onto her as soon as the woman sat down in the twirling waters. She was pretty and thirty-ish, with a voluptuous figure and long brown hair stacked on top of her head in a sexy, messy bun. Her soft, pouchy belly didn't detract from her prettiness. Susan left our chat abruptly, without even a "talk to you later," and made a beeline for a spot next to the woman. She moved so quickly that I almost got whiplash.

I later discovered that the woman was what the swingers call a unicorn—a single woman without a male escort. At Desert Institute, single men unaccompanied by women weren't allowed into the place. If they had been, the property would likely have been crowded with men. But a unicorn, so named due to their rarity in swingers circles, was welcomed in with open arms.

I imagine Susan had to move quickly before some other couple or individual grabbed the unicorn's attention. Susan's husband, an okay-looking Irishman about ten years her junior, joined his wife at the unicorn's side. He'd been chatting with other people in the hot tub while his wife chatted with us. He'd come over and join our conversation for a few minutes, then return to conversations started with other people. When he saw his wife making a move on the unicorn, he didn't hesitate to assist in the conquest.

I don't know what was said between the three people, but after very little time, their conversation turned to kissing and heavy petting. I watched with awe as they stood, their naked bodies dripping with water, stepped out of the spa, and headed into one of the hotel rooms. After about half an hour, they reappeared in the room that held the DJ and the round, red velvet bed, and began dancing. A male DJ was playing club-like music and disco lights bounced off the walls and ceiling. They danced naked and freely like no one was watching. But everyone was, including me and Ben. We had a perfect vantage point from the hot tub into the disco room.

• • • • ● • ● • • • •

The Institute reminded me of a line from my favorite TV show at the time, *The Walking Dead*: "we're all infected." I watched the show not because of the zombies; I wasn't interested in the undead. Rather, I watched because I find dystopian apocalyptic stories fascinating. I enjoy watching how humans behave when law and order vanish and they must figure out how to survive in a changed world that needs rebuilding.

In one episode early in the series, a main character named Shane was killed in a duel over a woman. Prior to Shane's death, people turned into zombies after being bit by a member of the undead. The bite would induce an infection that would kill the human, who would then turn into a flesh-eating zombie. However, Shane died by a bullet, not a zombie bite, and still turned into a zombie upon his death. It was at that point that the characters in the show realized they were already infected by whatever virus was turning humans into hungry zombies upon death. The phrase, "we're all infected," became the tag line of the series. That's all I could think as I looked around at the people at the Institute: "we're all infected."

I didn't exactly think they were infected with herpes, although they probably were. It was more of a mental herpes. These people all had *something*. I was at Desert Mountain because of the fear and low self-esteem brought on by my affliction, but I didn't know what made these people do these things. If it weren't for the fact that I feared losing Ben and facing life alone with herpes, I would never have visited this place. Were these people also inflicted with a fear of some sort? Did it make them feel young to be here? Were they experimenting? Were they trying to save their marriages? I don't know what their motivation was, but I knew we were all infected by something that drew us there.

Ben said he wanted to visit Desert Mountain two times per year, once in the spring and once in the fall, to "help clear his mind." He said that at the fuck fest, his mind thought of nothing else but the sights around him and it relaxed him. I could do that. Two times per year, sitting in a hot tub watching people be their most outrageous and amoral.

Despite the meditational benefits Desert Mountain offered Ben, I surmised that he also hoped the message got back to Deborah, through their kids, that he was still frequenting the club that they'd discovered together. Any time we went to Desert Mountain, Ben made sure to mention to Eli and Maddie that he would be going out of town to relax and unwind in Palm Springs. He didn't mention Desert Mountain Institute by name, but the reference to Palm Springs should have been enough for Deborah to deduce where exactly we were going.

I also secretly hoped the kids would mention our trip to their mother so she'd think Ben had found someone who could meet his needs.

Chapter 15

Our House

Ben's house was in the far north edge of the Las Vegas Valley in a newer development next to vacant land owned by the federal Bureau of Land Management. At least some of that BLM land would likely be released soon to be annexed into the city of Las Vegas and developed due to an ever-increasing demand for more and more housing. As less land was available within the central parts of the valley, developers were looking to the outskirts. It was happening at a rapid pace and new housing developments, such as Ben's, were popping up in areas that middle-aged, native Las Vegans had known as the boondocks during their childhood.

Ben's house was less than ten years old; it fit all of us nicely and still had room to spare, and he'd remodeled it to fit his needs and tastes. Yet he was ready to sell after owning it less than two years. The hinterlands had become the place to buy if you wanted a new, more affordable place, but Ben wanted to move back inland to the area where he'd lived until divorce made him a bit of a vagabond who changed addresses frequently. Most people fear change, but not Ben. The man needed constant movement.

His primary reason for wanting to sell and move was to be closer to his kids' schools. Maddie attended a private Jewish school and Eli attended a public magnet high school. Both learning institutions were fairly close to Deborah's house but far from where Ben lived in the north; when it was his turn to take them to school, he had to get up extra early.

Ben's second reason for wanting a house in his old neighborhood was so the kids could have friends over more easily. According to him, both Maddie and Eli had frequent visitors and overnight guests when they'd lived as a family under one roof because that home was close to their schools. Eli had a couple geek friends who drove and would visit him at Ben's house on occasion, but to get Maddie's friends to visit, Ben had to be the chauffeur. The friends' parents didn't care to deliver or pick up their kids from a house so far away, so Ben would pick them up and drop them off afterward to ensure his weird, unsociable baby girl had a social life.

Ben presented the idea of us buying a house together after our first anniversary had passed, but before we'd completed a year of living together. Despite the better judgment of my mom and sister, I agreed to his plan because he logic'ed me into it. Typically, he'd either steamroll me into following his plan with pressure to acquiesce or use common-sense logic to work me into agreement. This time his reason made sense to me. I agreed with him that, since we were heading toward forever together, there was no point in waiting to buy a place as a couple. I didn't realize until later that he also needed me as a cosigner or his plan to move closer to his children's mother and schools wouldn't work.

Ben didn't go backwards when it came to his homes. Each of the two dwellings he'd bought after his divorce were a step up from the last, and he was ready to not just move to a new location, but to move up. For a guy who hadn't earned an income—at least on paper—through his divorce, he found a way to finance big purchases. I admired his fearlessness and tenacity when it came to debt and figuring out how to get what he wanted.

In order to buy his current house, he'd borrowed a substantial amount of cash from his mom for a large down payment. The labor for his remodeling was financed by his clients; he padded his estimates for bathroom or kitchen work to include extra cash designated for himself. If he had a client who wanted new flooring, he'd use his negotiating skills to convince the client to pay a higher amount for the labor, which Ben paid to his Mexican crew on the condition that they'd do his flooring for free. Oftentimes I could tell by the Mexicans' attitudes while they were at Ben's house working that they weren't happy about the arrangement, but they were illegal and got steady work from Ben, so they let themselves be steamrolled as well.

Although he'd been able to stash away some cash since we started dating, he still lacked the proof of income to buy a bigger, better home. He needed me as a cosigner on a mortgage so he could get the more expensive place he wanted, which of course needed at least four bedrooms and a pool. He lacked proof of income, and I lacked sufficient cash for my portion of the down payment. But together we could qualify for the ideal home floating around in Ben's mind.

Ben came up with a plan that involved me signing him onto the title of my existing house as 50 percent owner, and when we bought our new place, he would pay the entire down payment, but I'd be 50 percent owner. We hit an obstacle when it came to who should inherit both properties if he or I were to die. Ben wanted his kids to inherit his half of both my house and the house we hadn't yet found but planned to buy together. To that idea, I said *absolutely not*.

I'd owned and paid for my house for fifteen years. Ben hadn't contributed a penny toward it and there was no way I was going to split any profit with his kids if he died. I had descendants of my own, two nieces and a nephew, and I didn't see why they shouldn't get 100 percent of an investment I had paid for. We were adding him to the title of my house to make up for his covering the down payment on our new house, not to enrich his kids.

As far as the house we were purchasing together, I disagreed that his kids should become 50 percent owners upon his death. We were both planning to pay 50 percent each toward the mortgage, and if he died, I'd be paying 100 percent of the mortgage. Or would I have to move out so the house could be sold and the profit divided between me and his three kids?

A lawyer helped us put in writing our agreed upon terms of survivorship for the two properties. If I died, Ben inherited everything. If he died, I inherited everything. I felt secure with this plan because his kids weren't involved in it. If he died first, I wouldn't have to deal with them. And if I died, I didn't care what he did with the property. Our deaths were so far off into the future, I figured, that we'd likely buy and sell several places over time based on the way Ben tended to move around, making this agreement null and void anyway.

In the case of a breakup, the single-sided piece of paper drafted by the lawyer stated that Ben would receive full ownership of the new house, and full ownership of my existing house would revert to me. I felt secure that I would have a place to go if worse came to worst, even if I had to rent for a bit while I waited out the end of a lease agreement that might be in place with a tenant. However, I planned to see to it that we didn't break up, as herpes would be the tie that forever bound us.

I hoped that once we bought a house together, his kids would go from seeing me as just another woman in the long line of women in their dad's life to viewing me as his partner for good. Maybe even Maddie and I could develop a friendship and talk to each other when she saw I wasn't going anywhere. I had a lot of hope going into this venture with Ben that our lives would merge and settle.

Our realtor and mortgage officer were both Israeli men Ben had worked with before, and most of the conversations about our financing and future home were conducted in Hebrew, even when I was present. Ben and the mortgage guy came up with the plan to make me the primary on our loan because my current house was an investment at that point and not my primary residence, and it worked to our advantage in terms of interest rates to make me the lead. Ben and the realtor communicated exclusively with each other, and I heard what Ben wanted me to hear about the process. I didn't mind that Ben was doing all the talking for us; I liked that all I had to do was follow along.

The first house we saw was too close to a busy street but the second one. . . man oh man . . . when we walked into it, we were both immediately smitten.

I'd fantasized about someday owning a house with a courtyard and this house had a beautiful one that went beyond what I'd imagined. It was lush with bushes; a huge pomegranate vine filled with fruit; a mature, skinny tree; and other vegetation. A balcony from one of the second-story bedrooms hung directly over the courtyard and looked like a marvelous spot to sit and enjoy a morning coffee. I thought how nice it would be for my guests to walk through this courtyard to my front door, admiring the lovely entrance to my home and wishing it was theirs.

Upon walking through the front door, Ben and I paused to take it all in. It was the definition of open space. The entrance area had a two-story ceiling, with two flights of stairs on the right going up to the second floor. All the upstairs bedroom doors were visible from the front door.

Looking straight ahead, our eyes were drawn to a formal dining area, which was joined by family or living room spaces on either side. The current owners, a Jewish man who owned a popular bagel bakery, his Mexican wife, and their eight-year-old daughter, had made the living room to the left into a gathering space for guests with a small, removable bar and furniture. The living room to the right was more relaxed and was obviously their casual family area where they relaxed in front of the TV. I could already envision Ben's black leather furniture in both spaces.

Out the back windows, you could see the resort-like, two-level landscaping in the backyard. There was a pool on the lower level with a slide reaching toward it from the second level, and an in-ground hot tub next to the slide. If you were sitting in the hot tub, you could see down into the pool and view the entire yard. Once we got outside to have a look, we found numerous fruit trees lining the side yard and big, mature trees in other places. The house's inside was beautiful, but this yard was my definition of perfect.

At just about 3,500 square feet, the place was gigantic by my standards. It was similar in size to Ben's marital home, but more than double the size of my North Las Vegas house. I never imagined myself living in such a big place. It had five good-sized bedrooms, three full bathrooms, a huge master suite with a large bathroom and massive walk-in closet, a two-car garage on one side of the courtyard, and a separate one-car garage on the other side. The stairway to the second floor was elegant and open, with wooden spindles leading the way up tiled stairs. The kitchen was perfect, with a double oven and huge island in the middle. It was so extravagant and so out of my league! Ben wanted it and would spare no effort in convincing me that this was the house we should buy. I wanted it too.

My mom warned that I could be putting myself in financial danger by buying this house and advised me not to do it. My Wisconsin family is very pragmatic, and their homes show that sensibility. My parents built a small house about twenty years earlier on land that had been pasture to the farm where my mom grew up. They'd bought a hundred acres from my mom's parents and built a place that was efficient, with three bedrooms and two small bathrooms. When Ben came with me to visit my family, which turned out to be every visit due to his belief that I shouldn't travel anywhere solo, he repeated his opinion that it made no sense to build such a small house on such a huge plot of land. But a small, efficient house was what was needed, not wanted, by my parents, and that's what they built.

Ben's fearlessness about overextending himself financially worked toward our favor and we put in an offer. The purchase price of $425,000 was above our $400,000 limit, but Ben told me not to worry. He'd find a way through the inspection report to obligate the owners to come down on the price, using his construction knowledge to claim that every little ding found by the inspector would be an expensive fix, and then we'd have leverage to amend the purchase agreement and lower the price. He was wrong though. The owner was also Jewish and, in my opinion, probably had as much negotiation in his DNA as Ben did. At one point, they stood face to face yelling at each other as Ben tried to re-negotiate the already negotiated purchase price and failed.

It was the first time I saw his hard-nose negotiation tactics crash and burn and I felt bad for him. I felt a little embarrassed for Ben that he tried to be a bully and was out-bullied by the seller. However, a few days later, the appraisal report was able to do what Ben couldn't. It came in at $35,000 lower than the purchase price, so we ended up getting it for $395,000.

Ben listed his house for sale and we began the process of cleaning it and making it ready for showings to potential buyers. Before I left for work each morning, I straightened everything, including the kids' rooms, and ensured the bathrooms and the kitchen were clean and ready to be seen. The kids, of course, weren't expected to help even though they were Ben's inspiration for moving yet again. As I picked up clothes off their bedroom rugs or cleaned their bathroom each morning, I'd think to myself that no good could come of creating such inconsiderate humans.

When the time came to move, Ben and I worked together to pack our belongings into boxes and cart them to our new place in our vehicles. Luckily his house hadn't sold yet, so we could take our time moving from the old place to the new. Each day on the way to work, I'd take as many boxes as would fit into my Sportage and drop them off at the new house. We transported the smaller stuff, while professional movers would soon take care of disassembling and moving the furniture.

I worked a full-time job and was using all my spare time to orchestrate the move while the kids had lives of leisure. Packing up their rooms themselves would've seemed a bare minimum of help, and taken so little effort, and it would also have quelled my growing anger at how useless they were. Of all the things they left in their room for me and Ben to pack and move—which was everything—it was their backpacks that threw me over the edge and led to a fight.

"Why couldn't you have at least asked them to take their backpacks with them to their mom's?" I yelled at Ben in disbelief and pure anger one day.

My memory has deleted the reason why they'd left their backpacks on a Sunday evening when they departed to start their week with their mom. My assumption is that they had time off from school and didn't need them. The thoughtlessness of leaving those backpacks, heavy with books, hit a nerve in me and made me worry about our future together. But for the fact that we had herpes, we probably wouldn't have made it past six months together, given my dislike for Ben's kids and his no-guidance-or-responsibility parenting style. As it was, I bit my tongue most of the time and soldiered on.

My friend Mark and I used to discuss the destruction divorced parents were causing the kids of America. Mark was a coworker during my time at the local building department and stayed my friend after I took a job with the state. I met him while I was married and confided in him about my many marital problems, and now he was my confidante regarding Ben and his kids.

Mark was twelve years older than me, with thinning hair that had turned prematurely white years ago, and no butt. He wasn't unattractive, but I saw him try to date practically every single female coworker at the building department and, it seemed, most other single women he came across. I found his willingness to date any and all woman kind of gross because it seemed to me he'd screw anything. But as friends, we were good. Lunching together was fun. I liked hearing his dating stories even though they codified my belief that the two of us would never date.

Mark was very similar to Ben in that he didn't like to be alone. He'd been married twice already and was working hard to find wife number three. He had the same habit as Ben of moving women into his home fast to try and solidify a relationship. Despite the fact that living together seemed to kill all his relationships, he believed merging his girlfriends and their minor children into his home after about a year of dating was an essential step to see if there was potential to marry.

Mark and I had no children of our own, but we were open-minded about dating eligible singles with kids or it would have been nearly impossible to date. We were also alike in our belief that divorced parents were destroying the world. Fear of the children choosing the other parent leads to undisciplined kids who are difficult for a stepparent to deal with. But in Mark's situation, he could escape his girlfriends' poor parenting and fear of her children through a breakup. He didn't know Ben and I had herpes and I couldn't just up and leave.

As far as moving to our new house was concerned, Ben said he wanted Maddie and Eli to leave his old house at the end of his custodial week and arrive at the new house at the start of his next custodial week worry-free, with their bedrooms in place. He wanted it to be a seamless transition for them. I was raised in a home with four kids and two parents who worked full-time; the kids in my family pitched in with responsibilities inside the home and outside in the yard. We even cooked for ourselves while our parents worked. Not Ben's kids—all food had to be ready for them in advance of their Monday arrival. Ben and I would spend Sundays shopping for their food, doing their laundry, and preparing food that would be available in the fridge for them to grab and reheat at will. All of this was done to ensure that they'd be free of responsibility at his house so that they'd never refuse to spend time there.

Despite all the effort Ben made to make their lives easy, Eli and Maddie couldn't be bothered to return the favor in the slightest of ways by taking their backpacks to their mother's house to help us move!

• • • • • • • • • • •

There were many times when the kids could've offered to help but didn't; it was just how they were being raised. Back when I'd recently moved into Ben's house, he'd begun the process of remodeling his master bathroom, and he and I were prepping the area for his men to arrive and get to work. Ben used a sledgehammer and his hands to rip the room apart and I took care of hauling the debris from the second floor to his pickup truck bed outside in the driveway. I made many, many trips up and down those stairs with heavy contractor's trash bags stuffed with sheetrock, fiberglass, tile, and wood. On each trip toward the stairs, I passed by Eli sitting on the couch in the loft family room, with his cat-ear headphones on, casually playing a game on his laptop. If he'd offered to help, I would've turned him down, but at least then he would've been excused to be a lazy bum without prejudice. To my disgust, he didn't offer. He didn't even so much as glance my way.

After we moved into our new house, Ben planned to demo the kitchen countertops to ready them for granite. He chose a weekend when Tyler would be home from college because, he said, Tyler could help him. I was out that morning for some reason, and when I came home, all three kids were in the formal living room watching a movie while Ben worked alone in the kitchen. I asked him why Tyler wasn't helping. It turned out he'd never asked Tyler to help; he just assumed Tyler would pitch in after Ben started working, which, of course didn't happen. Why would it? These kids were taught that it was ok to be pampered and lazy at Ben's house.

Coincidentally, the kids' mother sold her house and moved into a newly constructed development shortly after we bought ours. She bought in a fancy area that was still just a few miles from our new place and even closer to the kids' schools. When it came time to pack up her belongings and begin the shift to the new place, all three kids helped.

The boys even rounded up a couple of their friends to assist with the move.

Chapter 16
Israel Can Wait

B en had herpes outbreaks at least a couple times a year. A pain in his groin gave him notice that a blister or two were coming. I had a prescription for Acyclovir, a medication that, when taken daily, helps shorten outbreaks and prevent new ones, and I sacrificed my pills to Ben when his virus reemerged. He had no interest in getting a prescription of his own. I was consumed with fear about experiencing a repeat occurrence and took the medication religiously, which seemed to work because, unlike Ben, I had experienced no other reawakening of the virus in my body since my initial outbreak.

Between the two of us, we kept a sense of humor about herpes. The mosquito-borne Zika virus had just sprung up in poor nations around the world, causing babies to be born with small heads. I used to refer to my medication as my Zika pills because somehow it was less embarrassing to say they were for a virus that caused birth defects than to say it was for herpes, a condition that did little more than irritate you for a week at a time. The stigma of herpes was just so shameful.

Whereas my tendency was to let it get me down if I thought about it too long, Ben was upbeat and maintained that, if we were to have a sexually transmitted disease, herpes was among the best because it wouldn't kill us. Most importantly, my nerves were somewhat calmed knowing we were in this virus together. It was easier to suppress my shame knowing we both had it, and I'd never have to worry about rejection from another man because I was with someone who had it too.

For our first few months in our new house, Ben and I spent a lot of time together in the backyard clearing vegetation. I liked the wild look of many of the landscaped areas, with bushes and vines sprouting everywhere, whereas Ben liked a clean yard and was eager to cut away or remove any vine, bush, or tree that might drop its leaves into the pool. I often didn't see his vision when it came to the yard and feared he'd remove everything in the name of keeping the pool clean. I got my way on some suggestions to keep and trim plants, but we ultimately removed many because that's the way The Steamroller wanted it. Even though I would've left the yard as it was on the day we moved in, I had to admit that Ben's suggestions didn't destroy the lush look of the backyard and made it look clean and manicured.

When none of the kids were around, we would relax at night, naked, in the warm, bubbling water of our hot tub, and I'd look out over our yard at the palm trees and tiered landscaping in disbelief that it was mine. My home in North Las Vegas had a barren backyard. I lived in that house for years, with my husband, and it never occurred to Leo to use his leisure time or hoarded money to make our house better; he preferred to watch TV and nap. There were so many things I would've liked to have done to that house during my marriage, but with no monetary or physical help from my other half, nothing changed. Ben was relentless in his efforts to improve our living space, with constant upgrades and maintenance. I felt lucky to have found this guy, even if he came with herpes.

The inside of our house was regularly under construction: new tile, new carpet, re-stained kitchen cabinets, new kitchen countertops, a new bathtub in our master bathroom, a new metal banister to replace the wooden one, and on and on. Everything he did made the house look more elegant, even though many of the changes weren't necessary.

Ben was good about asking for my opinion when it came to selecting colors and styles for tile, paint, stain, etc., however the end result was always the selection he wanted. If I didn't immediately agree to his preferences, his usual persuasion tactic was to bring up a topic once, then let it go for a day or two, then bring it up again, only to temporarily let it go, and over and over during the space of a few weeks' time until I'd get tired of hearing about the subject and tell him to do whatever he wanted. And truthfully, I knew it would look nice in the end, even if it wasn't my style.

Just one of the changes he made hurt my sensibilities and I continued to think it was the wrong decision even after the work was done. As usual, Ben pushed me into doing what he wanted, which was to redo the front entrance courtyard. He took out all the lush greenery—the bushes, vines, and trees—so it could be a gathering space. There were plenty of other places to entertain and sit in the backyard and there was no reason for the courtyard to have been sacrificed such as it was.

Within a couple months of moving in, Ben's brother Elan, his sister Renae, and Elan's new girlfriend, Ina, came to visit. It was the first time I'd met any member of his family other than his kids, and they were immediately nice to me, which gave me hope that I could blend in with Ben's people. I took time off from work to entertain them while Ben continued with his contracting work. We shopped together at an outlet mall and the girls even attempted a hot yoga class with me.

Elan, who was in his mid-forties, was the oldest child in the family. He was an accountant who had recently started working with their mother in her established accounting business and would take it over at some point when the mother decided to retire. He was the better looking of the two brothers, with darker hair and skin tone, but he was short, maybe only a hair taller than me. He was supposedly some kind of tennis phenom in his younger days, while Ben was the musical brother who played the accordion and piano in hotel lobbies as a teenager. As an adult, Ben pulled out his accordion only on Hanukkah. His kids would scroll on their phones while their dad played a few songs before putting the accordion away for another year.

Renae was married to a diamond dealer, was in her late thirties, and had two small children under the age of five. Small like Elan, she looked in shape but smoked like a chimney. While her outside packaging looked healthy, who knows what all that smoking was doing to her heart and lungs. She worked at an accounting firm while simultaneously studying to be an accountant. She could've made her life easier if she'd completed her studies in her twenties, but she'd been a rebel who caused their parents many heartaches before finally getting her life in order. Ben hoped Maddie would straighten up in time like Renae had.

Ina was of Ukrainian descent, blonde, and skinny. When she took off her clothes and came into the hot tub in a bikini, I was shocked to see sagging skin hanging from her body. She must have been heavy at some point and lost a lot of weight. She also smoked like a chimney.

With her clothes on, Ina was very pretty and I could tell Ben liked her looks. He'd said how Russian and Ukrainian Jews had caused many divorces after they started immigrating to Israel in large numbers in the 1980s. The women were considered the epitome of beauty.

Even though the kids were scheduled to be with their mom the week their Israeli relatives were in town, I thought they would spend most of their time at our house to visit with their aunt and uncle, who'd flown across the world for a visit. Instead, they came over for dinner on their scheduled Wednesday but didn't spend the night. I found it odd that the kids stayed away since Ben wanted me to be so involved in their lives by cooking for them, going to their school events, and lounging with them whenever possible. My nieces spent a lot of time with me when I visited Wisconsin for holidays even though my travel was just from Las Vegas. But Eli and Maddie visited only briefly and Tyler didn't make it home at all.

Perhaps there was no urgency to visit with the Israeli contingency in Vegas because in a couple months' time, Ben and the kids would see them again in Israel. Ben wanted me to go on this nearly two-week trip he'd planned; however, when he was ready to book the tickets shortly after our move, I told him I was unsure how our new expenses would strap me financially and I couldn't afford the airfare at the moment.

I refused to let Ben buy the ticket for me because I said it just wasn't the right time for me, money-wise, which was somewhat true. Before moving into our house, I feared that each paycheck would go toward the house, and I'd have none left over for savings. We both deposited an equal amount of money into a shared bank account at the start of each month to pay for our mortgage, utilities, and food. I soon realized that there was very little strain on me, and I could have swung the trip to Israel. However, my true reason for not wanting to go was that I had no desire to make such a trip with Ben's kids.

We put on a good show for the relatives. Or maybe Ben and his siblings spoke about my poor relationship with the kids in Hebrew with me sitting there beside them, none the wiser. Later on, they would say they got the impression that the four of us—Ben, me, Eli, and Maddie—were getting along. I guess they couldn't tell from the little amount of time the kids were at our house during their visit that their mean little niece despised me and ignored me completely. In fact, if I were the only person in a room and she walked into it, she would quickly turn and leave.

I very much wanted to go to Israel. My siblings and I had attended a Catholic elementary school and I'd learned about Israeli cities during daily Bible studies. I'd never dreamed of visiting Jerusalem, the Dead Sea, and Bethlehem, to name just a few of the places that were embedded in my memory from my childhood days, until I started dating an Israeli. My hope was that Ben and I would make the trip to Israel together to check out his homeland and meet his parents and see his country . . . but without the kids.

I was glad when Ben and his children left for Israel without me because I'd have two weeks to myself without having to cook or clean for anybody other than me. Plus, my people were coming to visit. My mom, sister, and her two teenage daughters were going to take advantage of my empty house by spending a week with me in my new place. I couldn't wait for them to see how far I'd come from my little 1,400-square-foot house in North Las Vegas.

Despite my closeness with my mom and sister, neither of them knew about the herpes. Other than that big secret, I was a blabbermouth when it came to pretty much every other detail of my life with Ben, with the exception of the Fuck Fest. They knew Maddie hated me. They knew I thought Tyler was an entitled know-it-all. They knew I detested Eli's laziness. They knew I hated Ben's friends, David and Shuli. And they knew that I signed Ben on to the title of my house in exchange for ownership in our joint house, and they weren't happy with my decision. It would have been so much easier if I'd just told them I had herpes and that fear was the basis of all my decisions since I met him.

My mom and sister thought Ben was a slickster who had me under some kind of spell. Mom, who tends to go negative when she can't understand why people do what they do, was worried about what would transpire, materially speaking, if Ben and I broke up. I'd blabbed to them, of course, that Ben had wanted his interest in my house to go to his kids if he were to die, which made them wonder at his ulterior motives. Mom felt that Ben's people were not my people, and if our relationship went sour, I was going to be in a bad spot somehow, someway.

Chapter 17

Our Home, Their Life

I was hoping I'd feel more at ease in our new home than I had in the other one since I co-owned it and it was my dream house. But given that Ben's parenting accompanied us to the new house, it was hard to feel completely comfortable; the kids were still treated like royalty. Because Ben was my partner, I continued to help him do everything for the kids—grocery shop, cook, and clean—to which they expressed not even an ounce of gratitude. I navigated as best I could, avoiding any discipline but drawing a line when I could do so privately.

When we moved in, Eli wanted the bedroom with the balcony overlooking the front entrance courtyard. I objected to Ben behind closed doors because if that were to be his room, we wouldn't have routine access to the balcony, where I hoped we'd sit in the mornings and have our coffee. If Eli decided to sleep in until some ungodly daylight hour, we'd have had to fit our access to the balcony around his sleep schedule. Ben agreed with me and told Eli to pick one of the other two bedrooms up for grabs.

Eli selected the solo downstairs bedroom, which was a good choice considering it had a full bathroom with a walk-in shower next to it. Unlike the two bathrooms upstairs, it hadn't been updated; the shower was a prefab plastic enclosure with a cost-effective sliding glass door and cheap amenities compared to the rest of the house. It was very clean and nice, but Ben assured Eli that he'd upgrade it soon. Eli didn't have to clean it—I did—so he had nothing to complain about while he waited for his father to design and install a fancy bathroom to match the rest of the house.

Maddie's bedroom would be the second largest room, upstairs and adjacent to a full bathroom with dual sinks in the vanity, a separate room for the toilet, and a walk-in shower the previous owners had graciously upgraded before our arrival. Ben had picked this room for her because he planned to one day create an entrance from her room to the bathroom so she wouldn't have to be bothered to walk out her bedroom door and around the corner to the toilet. She was the youngest and would be living with us the longest, therefore she would get an en suite bathroom to make her already pampered existence even more pampered.

Tyler, who wouldn't even see this house for a few months after our move-in date, got the last room available by default. It was furnished just like his room at Ben's previous house, except the two extra mattresses against the wall hadn't made the transition to the new house. I convinced Ben that it made no sense to have these extra mattresses for guests when we had so many rooms for visitors to use already, plus we had four couches downstairs that people could crash on if need be.

I never imagined we'd have so many people staying in our house that we'd fill up all the rooms and maybe even the couches too; I just wanted the mattresses gone. However, that vision of our house filled with sleeping bodies strewn all over almost became a reality when Tyler asked Ben if he could bring five kids from school to stay at our house while they went to Electric Daisy, a week-long techno music festival held on the ground of the Las Vegas Speedway. There would be ten kids total, with the other five staying at his mom's.

While Ben typically indulged his kids, this request from Tyler was too much, so he said no—like me, he didn't want our place to be a college kid crash pad. With our place unavailable as an option, the kids' mother allowed her home to become a camp for those wayward youth. Deborah also allowed the kids—all eleven of them—to pile into her Suburban each night and drive to the concert grounds at the racetrack. A Suburban is rather large, with a seating capacity of seven or eight, but eleven required a lot of squeezing and stuffing bodies in illegally for all to fit. Even Tyler said only their "crazy" mother would allow kids to squish themselves into her personal vehicle to head to a concert. There were cops all over that area and who knows how Tyler wasn't pulled over for all the kids crammed in like a clown car.

Deborah was a licensed family therapist trying to build a business as a life coach. Allowing eleven college kids to take her car and drive it to a huge party didn't seem like what someone providing professional life advice should be doing.

I'd never met Deborah, although on Facebook I saw that she was a pretty woman whose marketing photos were heavily doctored but nicely done. I saw her regularly at the kids' school events and she made her presence known with constant trips to our house to drop off one thing or another for the kids, especially for Maddie. Her black Suburban would pull up outside our house, Maddie would run down the stairs to the vehicle waiting outside, then run back to her room with whatever her mom brought her, without a word spoken.

Deborah made no effort to introduce herself to me, nor did I attempt to introduce myself to her. Ben said there was no reason for us to meet. He hated her more than any other person on Earth, he proclaimed, and I was happy to support him in that feeling toward his cheating ex-wife.

Ben and I used to lie in bed and look at her life coaching Facebook page, which was open for the world to see, and mock her posts. One was a glowing review of her father and the role he'd played in guiding her to the financially successful life she proclaimed to be living. According to Ben, she used to complain often that her father treated her unfairly when she worked for him. When she closed real estate deals she'd gotten because of his business, he rewarded himself by taking chunks of her commissions. Based on her Facebook posts, you'd never guess that she'd ever cried to her then-husband about her father being a dick to her. But those past feelings toward her father didn't fit the narrative she was trying to create of being a successful woman who other women should pay to learn the tricks she supposedly cultivated on her journey to riches.

· · · · ●·●· · ·

Tyler didn't get to turn our house into a crash pad, but we had an aspiring party organizer at home in the form of Eli, who invited every nerd he could find to our house. Sometimes a couple would show up, sometimes a few. It didn't matter how many—none of them cleaned up after themselves.

It angered me to come home from work to find a few, or several, nerds splayed out playing video games and chowing on pizza and cookies, as I knew they would leave a mess. I was glad Eli had friends, and I wouldn't have minded them in my house, but Eli seemed to take pride in letting them be pigs like he was. They left everything for the adults to clean up.

Maddie was just as bad with her friends. One time at Ben's house, after Ben and I had gone to bed, Maddie and two of her pals made cotton candy with a little plastic machine stored in his pantry. When we woke up in the morning, we found sticky sugar and cotton candy residue all over the kitchen. Ben silently went to work cleaning it up. I asked why in the world he wouldn't ask her to clean the mess she'd made. He gave some sort of answer about wanting his kids to be free and have fun. Cleaning up after his kids didn't give me a sense of freedom or fun.

I looked forward to the day his kids were adults living on their own. We had our best days when they were with their mother. I was bound to him by herpes, not by his kids. All I had to do was shut up, grin and bear it, and wait it out until they were adults, gone and living on their own.

Chapter 18

Cats

Of the two cats I owned when I met Ben, my little six-pound black cat, Kitty, was my favorite. She was three years old when I got her and was the best cat I ever had. Except for the one time she used a carry-on suitcase as a toilet, due to accidentally being locked inside a closet all day while Leo and I were at work, she was a prolific litter box user. Every night like clockwork, soon after I'd settled in under the covers, she would jump onto our king-sized bed and snuggle into me as I lay in the fetal position. She was a good substitute for the husband who stayed up late watching porn.

My white cat, Boris, was harder to love. I took him in when he was about five and had been a stray. Soon after I got him and realized he was peeing on the carpet, I called around to local cat rescues to try and offload him on someone else. Unfortunately for us, and fortunately for Boris, rescues were full. I ended up keeping him, hating him from time to time, and investing in a carpet shampooer.

Shortly after moving into Ben's house with both my babies, I noticed that Boris didn't look well. My cats were about eighteen years old at that time. Even though Boris still had an enormous belly, I could see his backbone protruding from his shaved skin as if he'd been starved, but that boy never missed a meal. The vet diagnosed him with a slew of problems including diabetes, kidney disease, and a thyroid condition.

Boris lasted just a few months before I made the decision to put him down. He'd spent his last night wandering from the kitchen to our bedroom sneezing blood about a foot high on the walls. It looked like a massacre had taken place near the floorboards. The vet said he likely had grown a mass in his nose that had ruptured and could not be removed because of the small nature of a cat's nasal cavities.

It was the first time I'd ever euthanized a pet. I was in the exam room when the vet administered the fatal injection, and when his head drooped in death, I started crying and was overwhelmed by the feeling that I had murdered my cat.

Kitty lived almost exactly one month in our new house before I noticed something was terribly wrong with her. After a couple of days of secluding herself and not eating, drinking water, or using the litter box, I took her to the vet only to find out she had cancer everywhere in her body. Like Boris, she went into the vet clinic alive, and her life ended on that final visit.

With both my cats deceased, I wanted to go to the shelter to pick out a new one. Ben wasn't completely on board because he worried Eli, who hadn't been bothered by two cats, would have an allergic reaction to a new cat due to Eli's belief that he was allergic to *some*, but not all cats.

As happened frequently when it came to his offspring, Ben came up with a stupid solution to bridge the gap between what I wanted and accommodating his kids. It would have been so much easier to allow the adults in the house to make decisions, but his fear that any inconvenience, no matter how minor, would result in his kids choosing their mother's home over ours, took precedence over common sense.

In the matter of the new cat, Ben suggested that he, Eli, and I go to the animal shelter together, with Eli determining which cat I could adopt by holding each one to see if the cat caused him nasal congestion. I would pick out a cat I liked, but it was up to Eli to decide if the cat was acceptable or not. It was a stupid, unnecessary scenario and I wanted nothing to do with it.

Eli's belief in his cat allergy was due to a stuffy nose he experienced once upon a time while visiting a friend with a pet cat. I'd read an online article explaining that people with a loony belief in sporadic cat allergies were probably reacting to a pollen the cat likely dragged in from outside. Eli had seasonal allergies, which he treated, when in the mood, with a nasal saline rinse. It seemed logical to me that pollen on the cat's fur was the culprit behind the plugged nose he experienced *that one time* at the friend's house.

One Friday evening when the three of us—Eli, Ben and I—were in the car on our way to Ben's favorite Mexican restaurant, Ben divulged his solution to the cat problem. From the back seat, Eli seemed amenable to the plan to select my cat for me. I attempted to reason with Eli that pollen was likely the cause of his one-time allergic reaction to a cat. Eli wasn't amenable to my logic. He was allergic to some cats and that was the end of the story. What followed was a very silent dinner at the Mexican place. I was mad at Eli, and both Eli and Ben were mad at me.

Later that evening when we were back at home, Ben admitted to me that a blood test a few years earlier had confirmed that Eli was not allergic to cats. It was pure fantasy that some cats caused him to suffer from nasal congestion. In all the discussions Ben and I had had about cats, including bringing my two elderly cats into his house, he'd never mentioned that Eli had received this test. The results should have been enough to shut down the discussion once and for all, but instead, Eli's allergy fantasy, just like his irritable bowel fantasy, was indulged.

At least for the time being, I gave up my fight for a new cat.

Chapter 19
Who Needs Dreams?

I knew that if I never pursued a writing career and published a book, I'd regret it on my deathbed. I would start writing short stories and book ideas many times throughout my life, only to procrastinate and justify putting aside my writing to help someone else chase after *their* dreams. If I put my effort into helping Leo get his dental laboratory up and running, for instance, nobody would blame me for postponing work on my own dream. Now that herpes had been added to the mix and I felt bound to Ben, there was even more postponing. Writing takes a lot of alone time, which was something I didn't have much of with Ben. I was willing to feel some regret at the end of my life rather than deal with the solitude I was convinced I'd experience if we broke up.

I justified giving up on myself by thinking of all the people who'd died before me without achieving their dreams. Why should I be different from them? I had to get through this life with the hand I'd been dealt—herpes. God would understand why I failed. Besides, I reasoned, I had a nice house, and I could see wealth in my future if I stuck it out with Ben. What did I have to complain about? I was getting a lot despite what I'd given up, and I'd never have to suffer the shame of admitting to anyone, from family and friends to any other man, that I was damaged.

I had to be part of everything Ben did—that was our dynamic as a couple. He liked it that way and it was my tendency to help my partner. For his contracting business, I'd pick up architectural plans for him at the printer, go to the building department to drop off paperwork, or stop by one of his worksites before work to open the door for the workers. I even went to court with him when he was being sued by a client who paid a deposit and then changed his mind and wanted his money returned. Whatever Ben needed, I was there for him, whether it was moral support or grunt work.

If we had spare time on a Saturday afternoon, I felt a sense of relief that we had nothing to do, and my time could be spent painting or maybe even just relaxing any way I wanted to. Ben would thwart those plans because if I had free time, that meant so did he, and free time was something he didn't like. Maybe his thoughts disturbed him, and he had to keep busy to keep from thinking. I don't know what went on in his head; I just know that always needed to be doing something. We'd end up going to Chinatown for a cheap couples massage, going out for pizza despite me eating a low-carb diet, or he'd find people—other than David or Shuli, at my urging—for us to hang out with.

Free time on a Sunday was harder to come by because the last day of the week was spent cleaning, food shopping, and cooking to make sure Eli and Maddie's arrival on Monday, as well as their stay for the week, was worry-free. Sometimes Ben and I shopped together, and often I shopped alone if Ben was in the middle of a remodel job he needed to complete. Getting food for the kids meant not just going to a regular American supermarket, but also stopping by specialty kosher stores to find the Israeli junk food the kids expected to be stocked in the pantry.

Ben wanted my maternal instinct to kick in and for me to give myself selflessly to his kids. However, the effort I put into preparing for the kids was specifically to help make Ben's life easier. He worked hard to provide a good life for his loved ones, including me, and I figured the least I could do was take some of the burden off him inside the house. There were duties I would do without much complaint, such as cleaning and grocery shopping, because those activities benefited all of us. I had a harder time pitching in to prep super unhealthy meals or do their laundry.

Eli's "sex sheet," in particular, disgusted me, and I refused to pick it up from the top of the washing machine, where he'd leave it to be washed. He'd found himself a little nerd girlfriend, Victoria, and had developed a post-sex pattern. After having sex with Victoria, he'd take the fitted sheet from his bed and place it on top of the washing machine for someone else to take care of, because the little stud couldn't be bothered to wash his own soiled linens.

Victoria stood about five feet tall and weighed 100 pounds. With straight brunette hair that hung limply to just below her shoulders, she wore glasses and had two discolored front teeth that looked half dead. Her petiteness made her cute in a way, but clean hair and capped front teeth would've done her a world of good in the looks department.

Her parents, a White father and Hispanic mother, were divorced. Victoria and her younger brother lived primarily with their mother, who had remarried and cared for her elderly Mexican grandmother in the home. According to Eli, the mother and grandmother didn't like him because, he said, they were Mexican and Catholic, and he was Jewish. However, their dislike of Eli and his faith, if it were true, was probably due to Victoria's proclamation rather early on in their relationship that she would abandon Catholicism and convert to Judaism if she and Eli were ever to marry.

For childbearing reasons, she would have to convert because Judaism is passed down from mother to child. If she remained a Catholic, any child she bore Eli, despite his Judaism, would not be considered Jewish. I found it rather odd that she would convert so easily considering the fact she identified as a proud Catholic, and if you referred to her as Christian, she called that moniker insulting because, she said, "Christians don't have a tradition, but Catholics do."

I wanted to know how a person could go from being so proudly a believer in Catholic traditions to ultimately denying Jesus as the son of God, which she'd essentially be doing if she were to convert to Judaism. I never asked for an explanation, though, as I wasn't particularly interested in hearing her teenage logic.

This was the girl who was helping Eli defile his sheet. Ben and I joked about how the sex they were having was so dirty that Eli felt the need to remove the sheet from his bed immediately after. We concluded that the kids must be using the pull-out method for birth control and that Eli's jizz was spewing all over the sheets, which was even more reason for me not to touch them.

Ben said Eli hadn't come to him to ask for condoms, he didn't know if they were being used, and he wasn't going to ask because he said it was Eli's business. When Tyler came to Ben at fourteen and said he wanted condoms so he could sleep with his fifteen-year-old girlfriend, Ben bought them for him and said not a word when the two teens did it at his house. He had kept Tyler quietly supplied with endless prophylactics when Tyler requested them. Had Eli made the same request, Ben would've bought them for his youngest son as well, but because Eli was silent on the matter, so was Ben. However, Ben did help by dutifully washing that stupid sheet.

The condom question answered itself while at dinner at BJ's Brew House with just me, Ben, and Eli. Eli stated that he'd been banned from Victoria's house because her mother discovered that the two teenagers were having sex. Victoria had let the cat out of the bag by throwing a used condom in the bathroom trash bin rather than flushing it down the toilet to get rid of the evidence. It was apparently more than just Eli's Judaism that Victoria's matriarchs didn't like.

I questioned Ben about allowing Eli and Victoria to engage in sex at his house, and later ours, when Victoria's mother clearly didn't want her daughter participating in such activities. Ben said he didn't care what Victoria's mother wanted; he wasn't going to interfere or put a stop to it. I thought it was rather rude that Ben didn't take Victoria's family into consideration in the least, but I thought it was even ruder that Eli didn't have the decency to take care of his jizzy sex sheet.

I tried to reason with Ben that if Eli was old enough to have sex, he was plenty old enough to wash that sheet. One day Ben approached me and said that he'd solved the problem. He asked Eli to put it inside the barrel of the washer rather than on top, and I, therefore, wouldn't have to touch it. Problem solved!

The jizzy sheet would be out of the way, but I remained confounded as to why Ben didn't simply ask Eli to wash it himself. Why on earth couldn't he require any sort of responsibility from his children? Washing a sheet once a week (we knew this was the frequency of their sexual activities, due to the sheet's appearance on top the wash machine) would not even be particularly taxing!

At one point, a towel began to accompany the sheet inside the barrel of the washer. At first Ben and I made a game of guessing what they were doing with the towel and why it also needed to be washed. I asked him why he didn't just ask Eli, but for some reason questioning the goings-on between Eli and Victoria wasn't an option. Maybe it was too much an invasion of Eli's privacy, even though expecting me to touch that gross sheet—and now towel—was an invasion of my sanity.

The towel mystery was solved one day when Ben returned home earlier than expected and saw Victoria walking from the bathroom to Eli's bedroom in the same towel that eventually made its way to the washer with the sex sheet. Eli had no problem placing all his dirty underwear, socks, and clothes in his laundry basket in his closet, but for some reason the sheet and towel were too disgusting for Eli to wait until Ben got around to grabbing his laundry basket for Sunday washing. Both were so dirty in Eli's eyes that they needed immediate laundering. But not by him. Anybody but him.

I was raised so differently from these kids; watching Ben pamper them made me cringe with every fiber of my being. I tried to reason with Ben that laundry was the easiest of chores Eli could do for himself, but Ben would hear nothing of it. He wanted his kids to be carefree and that was the end of the story.

My ex-husband had been also waited on hand and foot all growing up; he was raised by his paternal grandma, who did all the cooking and cleaning, requiring no help from Leo. There were other factors in Leo's past that made him a bad husband, but this lack of household responsibility as a child no doubt contributed to him ending up a lazy husband. I wondered if this was the road Ben's kids were heading down as college roommates or married adults and hoped somebody—in a dorm room or in matrimony— would refuse to tolerate the laziness and put an end to it.

One evening, Eli, Maddie, Ben, and I were sitting around our backyard firepit making s'mores and chatting. As usual, Maddie acted like I didn't exist, as if I were a ghost, and directed her commentary only toward her father and brother. Eli nonchalantly made the statement that he and Maddie were lucky not to have any responsibility. He compared his life to his friends, who were required to do household chores, and a couple held part-time jobs. He was disgusted by the work his few friends had to do and I was disgusted by his admission that he was a lazy ass and liked it.

My blue-collar father and mother grew up on farms and imparted to their four children the value of pitching in and working. If my parents said we had to do a chore, we didn't have the option to refuse it. But then again, my parents didn't divorce and had no fear we'd choose one parent over the other. Even if they had divorced, I had no doubt my no-nonsense parents wouldn't have allowed their children to rule either household.

Every summer, my parents grew a couple acres of strawberry plants and would sell the berries for extra income to anyone who wanted to come and pick them, or the customers would pay us to pick the berries for them. All four of us kids were required to pick strawberries to fill orders. I'd grown an affinity for soap operas one summer and spent a lot of time being a "couch potato," as my father said. When an order came in, I didn't have the luxury of waiting for my program to end; I had to get up and pick strawberries.

One of the jobs I hated as a child was picking eggs from the chicken coop. The chickens were mean and pecked at my legs as I walked toward the cubbies where the birds laid eggs. My hands met the same painful fate as I stuck them under the chickens' breasts to retrieve the eggs being kept warm with body weight. I did it fearfully and without sympathy from my parents. It was a job that needed to be done and they made me do it.

Maybe picking strawberries and eggs is something a city kid would never have to know. But eating and wearing clean clothes is a requirement for people no matter if they're urban or rural. From the age of nine or ten, my sister and I would do the laundry for my entire family of six just so our parents, both of whom worked full-time jobs, wouldn't have to. All four of my siblings fed ourselves and each other when we were hungry by making a pot of mac and cheese or our version of hot dish, a concoction of macaroni, tomato juice canned by my mom, and ground beef. I didn't understand the logic behind coddling kids, who needed to learn life skills like laundry and cooking for their own survival.

When Maddie was hungry outside of mealtimes, Ben would take her by the hand or wrap his arm around her shoulders as he escorted her from her bedroom, down the stairs and to the kitchen to check out the refrigerator and pantry for food options. It was the same scenario time and again, and even though he talked to her in Hebrew, I understood by her non-verbal body language that she didn't care for any of her options. Her shoulders were hunched in despair, and she looked down toward the floor in pathetic, starving agony.

Maddie was a picky eater and preparing meals revolved around what she would tolerate, which was generally prepackaged junk food, plain spaghetti noodles, chicken schnitzel made by her father, or chicken fingers from a fast-food joint. However, she would also inexplicably eat seaweed crackers and sushi, two foods I couldn't tolerate, and I was not a picky eater.

Most Sundays Ben would make a pot of spaghetti noodles and schnitzel to have on hand for Maddie and Eli during their week with him. I bought an Instant Pot pressure cooker to help with meal prep and was constantly looking for Jewish recipes, or recipes in general, for food that Maddie would approve of. I wasn't a prolific cook, but I attempted to make Shabbat dinners for the family on Fridays, and I baked snacks my Jewish household members could eat during their holy days.

I just needed to keep my head down and keep moving forward to get through this life. The kids would be all on their own some day and then I would, hopefully, have time to work on my dreams. If I never got around to living the life I wanted for myself, I hoped the pain of unfulfilled dreams on my deathbed wouldn't be too great.

Chapter 20
Party Organizer

There were plenty of details about Deborah that Ben hated, especially the fact that she cheated on him with a low-paid mechanic. Ben recounted much of this to me, things she'd said and done throughout their marriage, as well as after their divorce. However, there was one talent she possessed that Ben missed. She was skilled at—and enjoyed—entertaining and party planning. The worst part about my lack of party-planning ability was that I could sense Ben's disappointment in me for not sharing his ex-wife's enthusiasm and gift for gathering people for dinners and birthday parties.

Mothers know how to feed groups of varying sizes due to constantly throwing parties for birthdays, school events, and religious milestones such as bar mitzvahs or first communions. As a childless person with no party-planning experience, a gathering of even five people caused me anxiety. To make matters worse, no matter how much Ben wanted me to enjoy party planning just as his ex-wife had, I grew to hate it, and the feeling didn't subside with practice.

Leo was the least social person I knew. Next to him, I was a social butterfly, which was a joke because I was far from it. I considered myself an introvert who liked social interaction on occasion. Leo was socially avoidant. I'd wanted us to have another couple or two with whom we could go to dinner or to the movies, or perhaps even wander around together at an outdoor food or craft festival. Leo put the kibosh on that little dream. Making conversation with people he didn't know well was something he loathed. On the rare occasion we did go out with others, I did the talking for both of us and it was exhausting. He often critiqued the things I said once we were back home and alone again. He preferred that I went out to dinner by myself with my lady friends, which was what I happily did.

After eleven years of marriage to a man who was antisocial both inside and outside of our home, I got used to a simple, quiet homelife that I admittedly enjoyed. Even after my divorce from Leo, I did zero entertaining at my house. I worked on my painting and prepping for craft sales, and when not engaged in that hobby, I did elaborate and time-consuming embroidery projects. Both painting and embroidery were therapeutic and solitary endeavors that allowed me to binge-watch a lot of TV, which is what I wanted to do at that point in my life. Painting and embroidery made me feel like I was accomplishing something while also avoiding life with hour after hour of TV. My eyes and ears may have been tuned to the TV, but my hands were busy completing projects.

I had taken up embroidery as a suggestion from my mother, post-divorce, because I needed to occupy my time with something other than painting gourds. During that time of healing, I embroidered two full-sized quilts and was working on a third when I decided I'd spent enough time in mourning. I wanted to start going out and doing things and I, therefore, needed to attempt dating rather than sitting at home alone working on old-lady crafts. Two months after making that decision, I met Ben.

Ben and I had very different visions of how our homelife should be. He envisioned a busy house full of social encounters. I envisioned a quiet, peaceful sanctuary. I wanted to come home from work to solitude, where I could decompress in the backyard with a cup of coffee, or anywhere in the house without having to share my space with anyone but Ben.

At one point, Ben invited a family of three to stay at our house for several days while his company remodeled their house. They were in the middle of transitioning from Southern California to Las Vegas and had purchased a home just a couple miles from our place. Although Ben became friends with several clients and we socialized with them, he didn't typically invite them into our house for an extended stay. With this California couple, though, Ben saw deep pockets and investment potential, and he was working that angle as their host.

The husband, Richard, was Scottish with a cool accent and black hair that he wore long on top and slicked back. He asked if I had coconut oil he could use to moisturize his hair but bought his own when I forgot to loan him mine. Although Richard's vanity wouldn't allow him to divulge his age, he was obviously in his fifties.

Richard was attempting to build an acting career and often left his wife and daughter alone for days while he was off filming small roles in B movies. Neither Richard nor his wife Tiffany held a steady job of any sort, and the leisurely lifestyle they maintained was bankrolled by family money (his) and the sale of a nightclub he'd owned somewhere in Southern California. Richard planned to sell his single-story California house once his family was settled in Las Vegas, which would bring in a ton of money if he listened to Ben's advice to add a second story to increase its value by hundreds of thousands. Ben, of course, would be the contractor for the work in California.

Tiffany was a much younger, blonde, ex-pro-football cheerleader with a smoking hot body. She was in her late thirties, very personable, and Christian. A crucifix hung from a chain around her neck at all times. Her job was to follow Richard wherever he went and to take care of their two-year-old daughter, Mary, who was named for their Catholic faith.

Richard and Tiffany were nice people and I liked them. What bothered me was the time Ben insisted I invest in this couple, or any other couple he was schmoozing, for that matter. When I came home from work, Ben expected me to hang out with him and the California clients while they ate Chinese takeout or some other food from Styrofoam containers. I usually worked out after work and showered at my Pilates studio. After a day of being with people at work and then participating in a group exercise class, I wanted and needed time to relax and decompress, not entertain guests. I had no desire to sit next to the beautiful Tiffany with my soggy hair and eat unhealthy food; I'd get fat while she stayed thin and gorgeous.

I didn't hide from the guests like Maddie did. I acknowledged people, hung out for a bit, then politely excused myself to go about my business. Not all the time, mind you, like his daughter, just when I was tired and needed space. It was hard for me to comprehend Ben's disappointment in me retreating to my bedroom for a break when Maddie wouldn't make eye contact or chat politely with the guests. Ben made no effort to school her in proper etiquette—not even after the California guests commented on Maddie's rude behavior.

During my many conversations with Ben about Maddie's personality, he admitted she acted just like her mother when it came to treating certain people like they didn't exist. When Ben's parents visited from Israel during Ben and Deborah's marriage, they'd wake up early and sit in the kitchen drinking coffee. Deborah would enter to grab a cup of joe and retreat without so much as a head nod to her in-laws or a glance in their direction.

It was almost hard for me to believe Deborah acted so rudely because I saw her sociability in action at school events, where she enthusiastically greeted other school moms with hugs and happiness. Ben and I used to make fun of the cell phone video pep talks she posted on Facebook encouraging women to have strength and be successful. In my opinion, she portrayed herself in those videos as a woman with great social skills. But apparently, she applied them only when it was to her benefit to create an image.

When Richard's twenty-two-year-old cousin, Joseph, visited from Scotland, I took the kid on a hike outside of Boulder City and spent most of the day with him. I also brought Tiffany to my Pilates studio for a workout, and together, Ben and I took her on a hike when Richard was out of town on an acting gig. Still, Ben lectured me on the need to be more accommodating toward our houseguests. He was afraid my not eating dinner with them would make Richard and Tiffany feel uncomfortable. If you consider the fact his daughter was antisocial with 99 percent of the people in the world, his feelings toward my supposed unsociability were pretty hypocritical. He told me he wasn't embarrassed by her behavior, but he was clearly embarrassed that I needed some time alone when I came home in the evening after work.

· · · · ● · ● · · · ·

When Ben and I attended other people's parties, I would analyze what the women of the house did to prepare, and I'd try to absorb a little of their strategy. For example, Shuli had matching plates, silverware, and napkins for everyone, and her appetizers, side, and main dishes were homemade. She was fancy in her display, and her dinner parties were more of a fine dining experience. You got the feeling you were getting a treat due to the effort that went into prepping the party.

Other friends, such as Stephanie, had low-key parties. She'd been a client who hired Ben for a spa remodel, and he was working to try and convince her to open a second spa that he would, of course, also remodel. Stephanie was blonde, young, in her mid-thirties, with two small children. She didn't mess around with fancy displays or time-consuming preparation. Her party food was served on portable tables in the same plastic containers the food was purchased in from the grocery store. She served potato salad, pre-cut cheese slices, potato chips, veggies and dip, and other easy food that came ready to eat. Rather than gather at a table, her guests ate wherever they could find a place to sit. Her style was easier and, had I been in Wisconsin with my family and friends, I probably would've gone Stephanie's route. But in Vegas, with Ben's fancy friends, I felt obligated to be more like Shuli.

Organizing a gathering reminded me of my experience teaching English in Mexico. I wanted to put on a good show for my students and subsequently overthought my lesson plans and grew exhausted at the constant thinking and planning, which led me to hate the profession. Unfortunately, I approached hosting with the same unhealthy vigor. I thought too much about putting on a good show for our guests and would ultimately buy and prepare too much food. Worst of all, I would be a total bitch to Ben beginning a day or two before the event because I was an unwilling host and resented him for expecting me to be like Deborah.

For our first Passover in our house, which happened about a month after we moved in, Ben wanted to fill his eight-person dinner table with people. According to his divorce decree, Maddie and Eli would be with him for this Passover, making our table half-filled with four people, including me and Ben. He needed four more, and David and

Shuli with their two youngest kids fit the bill. He would've liked to invite more people and would've used portable tables to fit them all in, but luckily the Israeli people Ben knew seemed to stick with their own families when it came to Jewish holidays and declined his invitation.

I was head over heels with anger when Ben announced we would be providing dinner for David, the Great Chef Shuli, and their two kids. What the hell was I going to prepare for that judgmental woman? Up until that point, we'd hosted only one gathering as a couple, over Memorial Day, at Ben's old house with my friend Heather and her family. They were my people, and they were easy. David and Shuli were Ben's people, and they were difficult.

I made matzo ball soup and Ben made his signature dish, chicken schnitzel. Turns out we didn't have to cook anything for Shuli. That miserable snot ate only the six tiny food items that were part of the traditional Passover seder plate (that she herself had brought to contribute to the evening). Every time we went to her house, I felt obligated to be a polite guest and eat everything she put effort into making. But at our house she snubbed my soup and Ben's schnitzel and instead ate the seder plate items, which included a tiny bit of matzoh, a hard-boiled egg, a piece of lettuce, a smudge of some kind of fruit paste, a small piece of lamb, and a sprinkling of parsley.

All those items held some significance to remind Jewish people of their forefathers' 400-year enslavement by the Egyptians. The Jewish people at our dining room table went through the Passover ceremony, acknowledging each item on the seder plate and the significance it held, with all words being said in Hebrew while I sat and waited for that portion of the evening to end. It was bad enough that I had to make small talk with these people who Ben and I both didn't like, but who he'd invited into our home out of his desperate need to be social.

When that woman refused our offerings and only ate the little bits of food on the seder plate, I was livid, to say the least.

Maddie surprised Ben by participating willingly in the Passover ceremony. As was her usual modus operandi, she sat with her chair and body glued to Eli's side and spoke only to him and Ben. She ignored Maserati and her brother and every adult in the room except Ben, who was proud that she actively participated in the Passover prayers without having to be nudged or forced. She even laughed a few times and seemed to enjoy the evening.

After dinner, my toleration of Shuli and David was over. I went to my bedroom and stayed there. Eli and Maddie moved to the more upscale of our two living rooms and played a video game together on the TV. Despite being in the same room and watching, neither of our two child guests were offered the opportunity to play. Shuli watched the gaming from the dining room table. Of course, no evening would be complete without endless chatter, which Ben and David seemed intent on doing instead of calling the evening over and going their separate ways. They sat for a while at the table and then later took the conversation outside.

Later, when our guests had left, Ben chastised me for my rudeness. He was right; I was rude. So were his kids for not inviting the two other children to play their video game, although they received no admonition from their father, as I had. But I'd made my point. I was sick and tired of those people and pretending to be their friends. Shuli's snubbing of our food was the final straw; I would not fake my way through an evening in their presence again.

A miracle happened soon after my first Passover celebration: Ben changed his tune about David and Shuli spending time at our house. He reasoned that David might start questioning where the money was coming from for the upgrades Ben had already made to the house, as well as future upgrades he planned. The income Ben reported on his taxes and my government salary certainly didn't equate to the fancy house we lived in, and Ben worried that David might demand to audit his accounting paperwork to figure out if he was owed some of the money that was going into our place.

When it came to the check Ben owed David monthly for website work, Ben started leaving it under the mat outside the front door. Previously, the passing of the check, which had risen to $5,000 monthly over the course of two years, was an opportunity for the two men to sit inside for a while and chat over coffee. Perhaps David realized the only way he was going to make money off of his business partnership with Ben was to charge a ridiculous rate for his amateurish website work, which Ben paid religiously without complaint to keep David out of his accounting books. Now the swapping of the monthly payment was a simple business transaction that David completed by lifting the mat, taking his pay, and leaving.

Ben also said he didn't want David around any of his clients, especially Stephanie and her husband, Jason, or Richard and Tiffany. These people were Ben's marks and Ben knew, with opportunity, David would weasel in on his game. David had a way of making Ben's friends his own and Ben didn't like it.

I was absolutely OK with his explanations for not having David and Shuli over, because we did once and it was one of the most unpleasant experiences of my life. If I was going to have to be like Deborah when it came to party planning, I at least wanted some control of who the guests would be. Ben could use whatever justification he wanted when it came to leaving David and Shuli out of the equation.

Chapter 21
Real Estate

During our first summer in our new house, I mentioned to Ben that I needed a new hobby. I'd given up my dream of writing and being his girlfriend didn't allow enough time for painting and selling my gourd crafts. And besides the time factor, Ben thought the hours I spent painting weren't worth what I generated in sales. I thought a new hobby would help me feel like I wasn't just floating along being his sidekick. Rather than learn a new pastime that would give me no return on my time investment, Ben suggested I give real estate a try.

In all my years on the planet, which added up to forty-four at that time, it had never crossed my mind to be a real estate agent. Ben planted the seed and I became intrigued. All I'd have to do was pay for at-home study materials and take two realtor exams to get my license. Ben would set me up at his friends' Israeli-owned real estate brokerage and bring me buyers and sellers. The hardest part about real estate is finding clients and Ben was going to do that for me through his day-to-day activities, talking to his connections and remodeling customers. In exchange for his client-finding assistance, I'd give him a cut of any commission I made. It wasn't a bad deal and I accepted it.

Essentially, the setup Ben devised would be the same deal Deborah had as a realtor for her father. Although she was in the process of leaving real estate behind for fame and fortune as a self-help guru, she continued to work for her father until her big ship came in, just as she'd done the entire length of her marriage to Ben. Her father fed her sales and commissions through his business, and now Ben would do the same for me with his business. Her father took a cut of her commissions and Ben would take a cut of mine.

It took four months of studying to feel ready to take the realtor exam. They were four glorious months of spending time alone in my bedroom with my books rather than having to watch childish TV series or movies. Even though Maddie was thirteen, her father and brothers treated her like she was perpetually five years old, and the TV programs we were allowed to watch in her presence were childlike, with no nudity and minimal swear words. Nobody paid attention to what she was viewing on her phone though. Her social media and YouTube interests were probably more adult-themed than the stupid shows and movies we watched if she were in the audience.

When I finally felt ready to take the state and national real estate exams, I passed both on my first attempt, on the same day. Ben said his ex-wife hadn't accomplished that feat; it took her two tries. I knew her only through stories Ben had told me that didn't cast her in the best light, but I felt like I'd accomplished something by being just a bit smarter, or, at a minimum, a better test taker, than she had been.

True to his word, Ben took the initiative to get me signed up as a realtor at his friends' company. Being a friend of a friend of the owners was good for me in terms of the treatment I received from the company's broker, Lydia, who supervised all the company's realtors and their transactions. She was a devout Christian and didn't downplay her beliefs in the presence of her Jewish bosses. She was heavyset, tall, in her mid-fifties, and had thinning hair she wore too long. She dyed it a maroon tint because she said it brought out the blue in her eyes.

Lydia took a liking to me, which worked out great in my favor. She could be gruff in her responses to her realtor underlings if she thought they were stupid, and she thought *a lot* of people were stupid. I turned to Ben when I had real estate questions and didn't rely much on Lydia for support, which probably made her think I was catching on quicker than I was.

Lydia told me often that she didn't have many girlfriends, and why she chose me to be her friend was a bit of a mystery. I assumed my connection to her bosses through Ben was her initial motivation, but more likely, my sympathetic ear drew her to me. I like stories and will allow a speaker to bend my ear for extended periods of time, and Lydia had a lot of stories and a lot of time to repeat them. When she called, I'd accept that I'd be on the phone for at least an hour while she talked and talked and talked. I'd put my earbuds in and allow her to go on and on while I continued with my government work, household chores, or whatever I happened to be doing at the time.

I tuned in and out of her one-sided gabfest and often lost track of the people in her stories; it annoyed her when she'd have to explain again who the people were and their significance in her life.

"I already told you this," she'd say with an irritated sigh. "*Remember?*"

She spun fanciful tales of events that seemed completely absurd and made no sense coming from a religious, buttoned-up, middle-aged woman. For instance, she claimed that while she was growing up, her father was in law enforcement and was strict, but somehow she unwittingly joined the Vagos biker club at the age of fourteen. After school she'd take her homework to the biker clubhouse and find a bedroom in which to study. Somehow her parents didn't notice her absence from home, and she didn't notice any criminal activity at the clubhouse.

The leader of the gang took a shine to her and protected her, she said. He gave her a ring she wore on her ring finger that signified she'd always be his "baby," meaning she wasn't his girlfriend, but she'd always be protected by him. When she wore that ring to this day, she claimed biker-affiliated people knew she was protected and would leave her alone.

She couldn't produce a reasonable explanation as to how she even ended up finding the clubhouse in the first place, or how she had so many male "cop friends." According to her, these cop friends would drop by her house for coffee and cake regularly, and they'd attend police auctions and purchase jewelry for her. When I asked how she came to know so many male cops, she said "through job interviews." She claimed to have a two-year degree in criminal justice and had interviewed for jobs in law enforcement despite not being able to take any jobs in the field. According to her, her name was in some sort of database for domestic violence victims, which somehow made her ineligible for employment with the police. I'd never had a job interview with someone who later became my friend after rejecting my application, and I didn't believe this was the case with Lydia either.

Lydia said her first husband beat her mercilessly and, even though it had been thirty years since they'd divorced, and they lived in different states, he still stalked her and, therefore, her existence was legally scrubbed from the Internet as part of a domestic violence program to prevent the ex-spouse from finding her. I knew that wasn't true because I Googled her and easily found her name, phone number, and home address, but didn't call her out for the absurdity of this or her other stories. I was fascinated by the fact that this grown woman believed anyone would find credibility in her tales.

Lydia's favorite topic was Greg, her current beau. He was more than a few inches shorter than her, with a fat belly and a long, scraggly beard. He'd been her roommate for a few months before securing his tenancy in her home by becoming her boyfriend. Despite her devout Christianity, she was living in sin with this man with whom she was totally mismatched.

As far as I knew, they were not bound to each other by an incurable virus. It appeared to be more of a situation in which Lydia needed to be loved and Greg needed a place to stay. He was a sovereign citizen who didn't believe in home ownership, bank accounts, or paying taxes. He liked the freedom to jump on his Harley and head to the California mountains to snowboard. He started attending church only after his relationship with Lydia began to falter and he needed to appease her.

His pattern had been to find occupancy in the home of a somewhat frumpy single woman and somehow, despite his gnome-like appearance, weasel his way into her heart. The relationships eventually failed when he proved himself to be useless. He'd move on to the next woman, whom he'd already begun to romance before his last relationship terminated, which is the scenario that set the stage for his tenancy and courting of Lydia.

Lydia attended church services and bible study regularly, and she preferred to sit home and crochet. She hated the outdoors and planned to never snowboard. No matter the huge detail that Greg was her opposite in every way, she appeared hell-bent on making a relationship with him work. She seemed motivated to be in a relationship—any relationship—rather than be alone.

Thanks to Ben's usual negotiating techniques, I had my first clients before the Nevada Real Estate Division had even issued my license. My first real estate deal would be a double whammy—I would help Jason and Stephanie, Ben's spa clients, sell their modest home and buy a big house with a pool and RV parking. Lydia said most new licensees start out helping a client purchase a cheap townhouse or condo. Those other licensees didn't have Ben pushing clients their way!

Ben wasn't only my client pusher, he was also my real estate trainer, which was supposed to be Lydia's job. I gave up 30 percent of my first three commissions to the brokerage in exchange for her tutelage. Because the Real Estate Division hadn't yet issued my license, Lydia was required legally to accompany me when I conducted any business with Jason and Stephanie. Ben made it a point to be present, as well, when Lydia and I showed them houses. When they finally settled on one and grew excited at the prospect of owning it, Lydia wrote up the offer and, with signatures, emailed it off to the seller's agent.

The seller and his agent didn't even bother to reply with a *no thank you*; they simply ignored our offer. I found out later that Lydia had filled out the offer wrong and suggested that Jason and Stephanie assume the seller's mortgage rather than acquire a conventional loan of their own. We deserved to be blown off for an offer so blatantly stupid.

Ben knew a lot about real estate transactions from having been married to a realtor and working at his ex-father-in-law's property development company. When Jason and Stephanie grew weary of the search for the perfect house to buy within their specified area and were on the verge of giving up, Ben knew exactly what to do to get them back in the game. He instructed me to find three homes outside of their targeted area that had all the amenities they wanted—big house, pool, big yard, and room for an RV. I found an area just a couple miles away from our house, where Ben thought they would get the best bang for their buck. He was right. My license had been issued at this point, and I was able to submit an offer on their behalf. The offer was accepted.

When the sale of Stephanie and Jason's existing house and purchase of the new one was completed, everybody got their cut of my commissions and I proudly deposited the rest of the funds into my savings account. Lydia convinced Avi and Ariel, the real estate company owners, to release me from training without my having to give them a cut of my future third commission because I'd done so well with my first two transactions. I was free from her tutelage, which I didn't need anyway because I had Ben.

Ben took an extreme dislike to Lydia and decided he was going to take it upon himself to get her fired. He felt she hadn't provided me with the level of service that warranted giving the brokerage, on her behalf, any of my commissions. He was right, Lydia's training lacked any true teaching about how to handle a real estate transaction. But I'd signed an agreement stating that I would be under her guidance through three transactions and I had no right to complain, especially considering she lobbied to release me after two. Still, Ben wouldn't let it go.

I was sitting at a barstool in our kitchen and Ben leaned against one of the counters as he placed a call to Avi, whose daughters attended the same Jewish school as Maddie, and spoke in Hebrew. When he finished the conversation, he hung up and told me I needed to call Avi to confirm that Lydia was a horrible trainer and broker. I refused to do anything of the sort. If his efforts failed to get Lydia fired and she found out about Ben's slander, and if I contributed to it, my life at the agency would be extremely tough, to say the least.

Ben was a bit surprised at my refusal to speak with Avi, and he was even more surprised when I told him that he'd embarrassed me. Since I'd been released from Lydia's tutelage, it was a moot point what had happened during my transactions with Jason and Stephanie; I was free to work with any new clients as I saw fit. The last thing I needed at my new side hustle as a realtor was for my broker to hate me.

When my commission check was ready and I stopped by the office to pick it up, Avi took me into the conference room to talk about Ben's phone call. I didn't confirm any of Ben's accusations or add to them. I don't know what Ben had said to Avi during their phone call, but I got the impression he'd made it seem like his complaints were mine. And truthfully, they were. But I didn't need my boyfriend to have that conversation and I didn't admit to anything. I listened to Avi's statements, thanked him for his time, and left the office feeling like a child whose parent had embarrassed her in front of her friends.

· · · ● · · ● · · · ·

Shortly after my first two commissions, I became my second client. I'd had to evict both my first and second tenants from my house in North Las Vegas and had grown weary of being a landlord. The real estate market had changed to the point that I would make a substantial profit on the sale, and Ben agreed to let me sell it.

Leo and I had bought that house for $130,000 in 2002. When we divorced during the midst of the Great Recession in 2011, the value had sunk to $80,000. There appeared to be no end in sight to Las Vegas' housing struggles and it felt like it would be years before the list price would rise to more than what we'd bought it for.

By 2017, however, the Vegas real estate market had changed drastically, and it made no sense to continue dealing with renters when my house's market value was now almost $100,000 higher than the original price tag. After all was said and done, I made a $120,000 profit when, after getting multiple offers, I sold it to a rough-looking, middle-aged couple from Nebraska. The Nebraskans were chain-smokers, and I felt bad imaging the future stains that were sure to mar every inch of my cute little house. But I felt damn good when I saw that $120,000 land in my savings account!

I immediately wrote a check for $40,000 to Ben. Our agreement was that after I sold my house, I'd give him half of the $80,000 down payment he'd made on our joint house. At that point, the agreement we'd had written up by a lawyer—the one stating that he owned half of my North Vegas home—was null and void. We now shared one property together and were square in terms of the cash investment we'd needed to buy it.

Ben was all too aware of the amount of money sitting in my savings account and wanted to find a way for me to invest it. I was all too happy to let it sit in the bank. He liked to say he was an "outside of the box" thinker; he wasn't going to let up on suggesting creative ways to invest my funds until he hit on the right one.

One of his ideas was for both of us to invest in a home that Tyler would rent from us upon his graduation from college and return to Las Vegas. We used my MLS subscription and license to start looking online for medium-sized houses near where we lived. Ben wanted Tyler nearby, and he wanted to make sure the rental would provide sufficient fun for Tyler with such amenities as a pool.

I didn't object to the fantasy of buying a rental for Tyler because I wouldn't have to deal with strangers renting the property, but more importantly, Tyler wouldn't be living with us. I was already outnumbered in the house with Ben, Maddie, and Eli. Adding Tyler, the know-it-all party organizer, to our household scared me a bit. I'd learned that buying a house with Ben did not raise me higher on the totem pole of importance—the kids were still on top, Ben in the middle, and I was solidly on the bottom. I looked forward to the day when all three kids were on their own, and if I could help them by providing a rental property for at least one of them to live in, I was onboard. And if Eli decided to move in with his brother, all the better!

To my dismay, it turned out the idea of buying a rental for Tyler was short-lived. Ben decided, with no consultation with Tyler as to his after-graduation plans, that it would be better for Tyler to move in with us. But Tyler couldn't just have a bedroom and share Maddie's bathroom. Ben's outside-of-the-box idea was to create a luxurious master suite for Tyler that would include an en suite bathroom for his use only. To do so, he'd need to reroute plumbing and take valuable square footage from Maddie's room.

Ben hadn't given up on the idea to do an en suite bathroom for Maddie, as well, and ideally, Eli would get one also. However, we didn't have enough space for four master suites, so it wasn't an option. Unless, Ben said, we bought a new, bigger house.

The pursuit of a bigger house with a bigger yard crept into Ben's head, and like all ideas he had, he fixated on it and tried to steamroll me into acquiescing to his wishes. Although I didn't buy into his idea, I found no harm in searching online and using my realtor's license to access and view a couple big houses. As we walked through one place he particularly liked, he talked about how he'd design the upstairs to accommodate his vision of separate living quarters for all. The pool in the backyard was fabulous, with a swim-up bar that he envisioned full of Tyler's friends. Ben finished that walk-through with ideas cartwheeling through his head and certain that his vision of the future could be a reality. I walked away fearful of what my future held.

I had no maternal experience to draw on, but I thought the object of raising kids was to parent them right and then release them into the wild. I wanted to live alone with Ben. I wanted to travel alone with Ben. I wanted to have dinner alone with Ben. I could understand how the trauma of leaving his kids at the end of his marriage made him want to bind them to him for as long as possible. I knew the trauma of being diagnosed with herpes and how I felt bound to him. But I wasn't bound to his kids.

He told me often that he was happy with me and that he wasn't a quitter. The problems I had with his kids and vice versa could be solved; we would figure it out as time went on. But this idea of his to create a living space the kids would never want to leave was too much—it made me sad and anxious.

Chapter 22
The Rings

For the third birthday I'd spent as Ben's girlfriend, he surprised me with a trip to a jewelry store in a nearby strip mall for us both to pick out rings. Even though his plan was to be married again within five years of his divorce, and he was awfully close to the five-year anniversary of splitting up with Deborah, in my mind these weren't engagement rings. I had no timeline for when our marriage would occur, and I was in no hurry to bind myself to Ben with legal paperwork in addition to herpes. But I wanted us to wear rings—especially him—to mark us as being committed to each other.

My birthday falls on Christmas Eve, which can be quite a bummer. I'd learned a long time ago not to expect much in terms of parties or dinner gatherings in my honor, not because people don't like me or don't want to celebrate the day of my birth, but because everyone is busy preparing for the big holiday the next day. Dating a Jewish guy whose religion didn't include celebrating the birth of Christ had no impact on my lack of expectation for my birthday.

Six months after we'd started dating, my birthday came around while we were visiting my family in Wisconsin for Christmas. At one point, he secretly pulled my sister aside and asked her if my family was getting a cake for me. If not, he wanted to give my sister money to go buy one. She told him my niece, Rilee, planned to make me a carrot cake, my favorite, and he was satisfied that I would be properly acknowledged. I was also satisfied, after my sister told me what he'd done, by his sweet and thoughtful gesture.

As luck would have it, my second birthday as Ben's girlfriend was not only on Christmas Eve, but also on the first day of Hanukah. I didn't mind celebrating Hanukah with my Jewish boyfriend rather than celebrating my birthday. His kids were with their mother and, perhaps because it was my birthday, he didn't push me to pretend to be friends with that weird and braggy couple, David and Shuli. Instead, Ben worked his magic and managed to get us invited to the home of another friend, Ehud, a married Israeli father of two young children. An Israeli neighbor, Moshe, and his wife would also be there with their two young children. I sat at the kitchen table with the other adults and read an eBook on my Kindle while the kids played in another room and the adults spoke in Hebrew.

I'd been married to a Mexican who only spoke Spanish when we met, and I would translate conversations for him so he would be included. But I was OK letting these Israelis speak in their mother tongue, even though they all knew English. It was somewhat awkward; however, I didn't mind reading quietly while Ben laughed with the others at unknown things that were said right in front of me in another language. I knew Ben was enjoying it, so I didn't complain.

By the time my third birthday came upon us, we were living together in the house we'd bought. This would be another year with all three of his kids under our roof for the winter break. We would have a nice lunch at the Cheesecake Factory, which I picked because it was where I wanted to go, and I was sure there would be chicken fingers on the kids' menu for the very finicky Maddie. We would tell the kids about our rings during the meal.

Women look at a man's ring finger to sum up the story of his current life; it tells them if he's available. I know it's true because I do it. Through conversation, they find out what kind of job he has, and thus his source of income. They look at the car he drives to verify if the story of his income is true.

Ben's income was progressively growing, and it didn't take him long after meeting someone to talk about money and his success. He'd spoken too openly about his possessions when he first met my brother, and it had been a turnoff. But women, on the contrary, are often turned on by a man's talk of his accomplishments and even more if he mentions his expensive possessions.

Ben spent a lot of time on the phone and at the homes of women discussing remodeling. I feared that, if the woman wasn't interested in Ben for herself, she might have a friend who she thought he should meet. I hoped these women would be stopped in their tracks if they saw the ring and knew their general contractor, who traded in his pickup for a new one every two years, and who talked ad nauseum about the expensive remodeling he'd done to his own homes, was taken.

I had no idea if any women would be interested in stealing Ben after finding out about his herpes status. Not that he'd necessarily tell them—he hadn't told me, after all. But perhaps by the time they found out, they'd stick with him, like I had done. He'd have a new lover and I'd be doomed to be alone the rest of my life.

It seemed obvious to me that Ben's standard of living and showmanship would lead a lot of women to put aside any fear of his sexual health status if they calculated all they could acquire by exposing themselves to his virus. Famous musicians seem to have a steady stream of gorgeous women despite having screwed half the world's female population and probably sporting the same virus Ben and I shared. Although I'd read only rumors of famous people with herpes, I guessed many had it based solely on the likely number of times they would've exposed themselves to it, with their incessant chase of tail.

Later that evening, with the new rings still fresh on our fingers, the five of us loaded into my used, but new-to-me Cadillac SRX, with Ben in the driver's seat, for the trip to the Cheesecake Factory. Ben had decided that my Sportage wasn't elegant enough for his taste and started his steamrolling tactics to convince me to trade up. His sister in Israel had recently bought an SRX and he decided that's what we needed to have as well. I used a little steamrolling of my own and refused to buy anything that would increase my car payment. He found the SRX he wanted at a local dealer, negotiated the deal and made a down payment sufficient to keep my payments the same as what I'd been paying monthly for the Sportage.

We unloaded from my SRX in the Cheesecake Factory parking lot and began the short walk to the restaurant. The two boys walked in front of me, and Ben and Maddie walked behind me. She'd already begun her pouting routine before leaving the house and, as Ben walked her toward the restaurant, he guided her with his arm around her shoulder and spoke to her in Hebrew. She walked with her head down and shoulders slouched, as if going to the Cheesecake Factory was a total burden on her little, put-upon self.

Ben called to me to get my attention, and I turned to look at him over my shoulder.

Maddie raised her head ever so slightly and, with her eyes still looking toward the ground, muttered, "happy birthday," in the most pathetic voice, forced unwillingly out of her body.

Ben gave me a pleased look. It was the same look he plastered on his face every time he got Maddie to acknowledge me with a half-assed, no-eye-contact greeting.

Ben spoke to her again in Hebrew. I assumed, based on her response, that he'd asked her why she was behaving like a whiny little baby.

"I have a headache!" she exclaimed emphatically and near tears.

This trip to the Cheesecake Factory on my behalf was likely to kill her. I didn't thank her for the rude acknowledgment of my birthday, and we all continued forward to the restaurant. I hated that Ben insisted on bringing the kids to our dinner when it could've been a nice outing with just me and him.

Once at the table, Maddie's headache persisted and she continued her pouting routine seated next to her brothers. Ben and I did most of the talking to each other as the kids entertained themselves with their phones.

Ben's announcement to his kids that we were wearing rings was met with a genuine lack of enthusiasm. I wasn't going to be their stepmom anytime soon, which was something the kids could have rallied behind. I didn't expect hugs and didn't get any. Not soon after the announcement was made, the kids returned to their phones and Ben and I to our conversation.

Just as we were about to finish our dinners, Tyler and Ben began to speak to each other in Hebrew. Soon after their conversation ended, Tyler slipped away from the table for what I assumed was a restroom break. When a waitress arrived with a piece of chocolate cheesecake for me in honor of my birthday, I realized Ben had asked Tyler to set up this surprise. The waitress brought enough forks for all of us and we shared the slice of cheesecake and it was nice.

Chapter 23

My Apartment, Part I

My apartment was close to work, one bedroom, and a perfect escape from Ben and his kids. During Ben's custodial weeks, I stayed at my place until the kids left on Sunday. I'd go home to Ben on Wednesdays when the kids spent the night with their mom. I was master of my domain in my apartment, sitting perfectly on the top of the totem pole with nobody underneath. While at the same time, with me out of the way at our house, Ben was free to parent how he saw fit, and the kids could rule the house without a pesky interloper watching everything and judging. It was a perfect solution to the problem of how the kids and I could coexist in peace.

To furnish my apartment, I'd limited myself to basic kitchen supplies and a few pieces of secondhand furniture. I saved money on food and gas by going to my apartment for lunch and walking to work. I even satisfied my itch for a cat by keeping one at my apartment.

Unfortunately, my apartment was just a daydream. There were three new apartment complexes going up near my office building, and each time I drove by any of them, my head spun with ideas of what it would be like to rent one for an escape. Just for fun and curiosity, I checked the websites for each complex to explore the amenities offered, lease lengths, and monthly costs. I calculated whether I could afford a rent payment in addition to my current household expenses. It would've been tight without dipping into my savings on occasion, but a six-month trial run would've been worth a shot.

This apartment idea had substance and could've been an interesting experiment. Unfortunately, Ben disagreed. He was shocked and a little hurt when I told him of my apartment fantasy. He couldn't comprehend why I just couldn't make myself happy. I had a big house, a gorgeous kitchen and beautiful master bathroom, both of which he'd remodeled, and I loved our backyard. Why couldn't I roll with the kids the way they were instead of getting angry and offended? If they didn't acknowledge me with a hello, or say thank you for a meal I made for them, or treat me as if I existed, why couldn't I realize that's just how kids were? Because that was a bullshit excuse for his kids' bad behavior and it made me dislike them, and I was growing increasingly resentful toward Ben for allowing it.

My relationship with Tyler was consistently fine; he was away at school most of the time and our interactions with each other were mostly superficial. Maddie's and my interactions were also consistent—consistently bad. After nearly three years, she still couldn't stand me; I knew that I was persona non grata in her eyes. However, my relationship with Eli, who was the most amiable of the three kids, took a turn for the worse after he graduated high school and started his first semester of college at the University of Nevada, Las Vegas.

I'd heard often that Eli was a smart kid when it came to computers, but I guess he just looked the part of a nerd because he wasn't accepted at either of the two California universities he applied to, including the one Tyler attended. His SAT scores weren't high enough for those places and he had to settle for local UNLV.

Eli was disappointed that his college career would be local, but Ben was ecstatic. The tuition costs at UNLV were far less than either of the two California options. Plus, Eli would continue to split his time between our house and his mother's rather than live on campus, which would mean no dorm or campus meal plans to pay for.

While attending college, Eli maintained his core group of four or five nerd friends from high school and his nerd girlfriend. She was one year younger than Eli and planned to go to community college after high school. She hoped to transfer to UNLV eventually. Her life plan still included converting to Judaism if she and Eli were to make it as a couple.

Eli often had friends over. Most of them were polite and would greet me when I got home after work, however I grew tired of them regularly being at our house on weeknights and entire afternoons on the weekends. It wasn't that I minded the nerd games they played on their laptops at the kitchen table; it was good, clean fun. I minded that the kids were loud and made a mess of the kitchen and dining area, where they played. And I minded that I had no indication there would be a group of kids at my house when I arrived home from whatever adult thing, like work or working out, that I had been out doing.

Surprisingly, Ben agreed with me that Eli needed to advise us of his gatherings beforehand. Ben came around to my viewpoint when an at-home massage he'd scheduled for a weekday afternoon was interrupted by hollering and screaming from the first floor. Eli and his friends were taunting each other in play while, on the second floor, a masseuse tried to rub the knots out of Ben's back. Shortly after the massage incident, Ben instituted a rule that Eli would have to advise both of us before bringing his troop of nerds to our house for entertaining.

It wasn't a hard assignment; a simple text to me, maybe a short call to his father, and Eli could go on with his plans. If either of us needed quiet in the house, we would let Eli know that any gathering of his would have to wait for another day. I had no plans to ever say no—I was just making a point that I mattered and that the adults of the home ran the show. However, after just a couple text advisements that nerd games were planned, to which I responded positively, Eli grew a disdain for having to ask my permission.

One typical Sunday morning, Ben and I were outside cleaning up the yard, pruning and doing yardwork, while Maddie and Eli were being lazy, doing whatever lazy kids do on a Sunday, inside the house. At some point, Eli was planning to leave to play Dungeons and Dragons with his friends.

Eli came out of the house and spoke to Ben in Hebrew. The two had a short conversation, and Eli went back inside. After he walked away, Ben informed me that Eli's friends would be coming to our house to play because the place where they were supposed to go fell through. I had no objection to the kids coming to our house, but I objected to Eli speaking in Hebrew when he could've asked us both for permission in one fell swoop, in English. He chose Hebrew on purpose to show me that what I wanted didn't matter, and that he'd get away with it too.

"You mean to tell me that he came out here, with both of us standing here, and asked you for permission in Hebrew?" I asked incredulously. "He did it on purpose to be rude to me." I gave Ben a look and shook my head.

Ben knew I was right; he went inside and came back out with Eli. After exchanging a few words in Hebrew with his dad, Eli looked at me and apologized in English.

And then it happened. All the feelings I had about the kids – the resentment that they didn't lift a finger, the frustration at their lack of gratitude, the knowledge that I was the lowest in the family hierarchy, all of it boiled over and exploded out of me.

"I don't give a fuck what you do!" I snapped.

My response was, admittedly, out of line. But anger had taken over and there was no stopping it. I could see by his wide eyes that Eli was surprised by my words. He turned and headed into the house without responding. I continued with the yard work.

Later that day, Ben and Eli had a private talk outside in the area where Ben and I shared our morning and evening coffees. Afterward, Ben shared that Eli had said he didn't like me, his nerd girlfriend Victoria didn't like me, and Maddie didn't like me either. I knew Maddie had disdain for me because she made no attempt to hide it. But the other two could be very personable to me and we had polite conversations. Admittedly, the childlike things both said agitated me, but I thought Eli's problem with me was that he didn't want to accept me as an authority figure in the house; I didn't think he disliked me.

Later that evening, Ben tried to broker a truce between us; he brought Eli to our bedroom, where I was already tucked in for the night, to talk things over. Eli and Ben stood in the doorway while I reclined in bed. I don't remember what Eli said, but I remember what I said as the two of us started screaming at each other. I told him he was a man-child and fake. If he was old enough to have sex, he was old enough to take responsibility for his sheets. I said the only real person in the house was Maddie because at least I knew without a word spoken that she didn't like me.

Eli turned from the doorway and left the house in anger with his sister, who had started crying uncontrollably from her bedroom, from where she overheard the argument. She could be the coldest, meanest little thing, but her feelings were also easily hurt, and she had a hair trigger when it came to crying. Worse than crying, she'd gotten into cutting her wrists with a friend at one point. For a time, she was banned from seeing that friend, but who knows if Maddie wasn't the influencer in that situation. There were obviously a lot of things going on inside that head.

After the kids left, Ben cried. His nightmare that he'd lose his kids to their mother appeared to be coming true. And for a bit, it was true, although it was temporary. Maddie came back in a day or two and Eli returned after a couple weeks.

That night I felt relief. I'd held in my thoughts for so long and it felt good to have gotten them out. There were many things I could've said differently that day that might have changed the trajectory of my coexistence with Ben's kids, at least in the short term. The way my words projectile vomited from my mouth wasn't ideal, but however I said them, the end result would've been the same. Eli's and Maddie's shitty behaviors hadn't gone unnoticed, and I let them know they were jerks.

Ben spent a few hours that evening calling Israel for advice from his mom, and California for advice from his oldest son. One of his advisors told him to hide his gun from me; he'd bought it a couple years earlier in response to a threat from two young, burly White guys who were doing tile work for him. He'd screwed them over somehow and felt threatened enough to buy a gun, which neither of us knew how to load or shoot, making it a useless weapon.

I was on the phone with my sister when I saw Ben with the gun. He told me he'd been advised to hide it from me, and my response was to laugh. My sister was of the opinion already that Ben and his kids were intolerable and wanted only to know why I couldn't break free from these people. I asked myself the same question repeatedly, but my answer was always herpes. I'd been given a life sentence that I couldn't tell anyone about for fear they'd worry I would contaminate their homes and toilet seats when I visited.

In the days after the big fight, Ben spoke on the phone to more family members in Israel and local friends, telling them about our troubles. He'd been silent up until that point and the people who knew him were surprised to find out we didn't have the happy household Ben so often proclaimed existed. He'd frequently tell me he was happy and that he wasn't a quitter, which must have been the same message he was telling everyone else. I was not so silent. My friends and family were well aware of my feelings toward Ben's kids and friends.

His mother, Miriam, advised Ben to implement consequences for the kids for their bad behavior. I'd offered the same sage words to Ben many times, but it took hearing that advice from his mom before he took action to try and correct his kids' mean behavior toward me.

· · · ● · ● · ● · · ·

Ben had planned a trip for the four of us to visit Tyler at college over Mother's Day weekend. Tyler's fraternity was hosting an award ceremony and dinner on Saturday evening at a fancy party hall, followed by a Sunday breakfast at the fraternity house that was to be prepared and served by the boys in honor of their mothers.

I insisted that the misery of traveling with his children just wasn't worth it for me and refused to go. But as it turned out, Ben and I ended up going alone. The advice he'd gotten from his mother was to tell Eli and Maddie that they couldn't go on this or future trips, including an upcoming trip to Israel, if they made no effort to be nice to me. They chose not to travel to see their brother.

The trip to California turned out just fine. Tyler was pleasant to me despite the fight I'd had with his brother and his sister's hatred of me. He didn't seem to hold it against me and was amiable.

A month later, during Father's Day weekend, Ben and I loaded up his truck and headed back to Tyler's college campus for his graduation ceremony. We had to take his truck rather than my Cadillac because the plan was to pack up Tyler's things at the finale of the weekend and bring them back to Las Vegas. Tyler had travel plans he needed to take care of, which was good because he hadn't decided if he wanted to live with us, his mother, or somewhere else. I silently prayed that he would move in full-time with his mother.

Eli and Maddie rode with Deborah and Wrench Boy to the ceremony and stayed with them in their hotel. As usual, Wrench Boy tried hard to cover his blue collar, mechanic background with a suit and tie. He outdressed Ben, who wore slacks and a polo shirt to the graduation ceremony. For the life of me, I couldn't understand why Eli and Maddie—especially Maddie—seemed to have no problem with the poser their mother hooked up with but were intolerant of me.

The graduation ceremony was held on the college's football field. Prior to the start of the ceremony, Eli and I came face-to-face on the grass in front of the stands, where family and friends were to sit and listen to the boring commencement speeches about life and the future. To his credit, Eli acknowledged me first. He said hello and I said hello back. Neither one of us apologized. From that point forward, my relationship with Eli returned to what it had been. The four of us politely engaged in taking photos with the graduate, dressed in his cap and gown, as if we were a happy, blended family.

The Maddie situation was a little more difficult than dealing with Eli because she was such a stubborn cunt. It didn't matter that Tyler had no problem with me, or that Eli and I had made up. She was determined to treat me as an outcast, and she was so damn good at it!

The language I used when I spoke to anyone about Maddie, including Ben, had grown horrible. I knew she was just a kid, even though she had the meanness of a bitter middle-aged woman who'd been abused her whole life. I was wrong to refer to her as a cunt or bitch even when I was in the safety of my friends and family, and even worse, when I used that language in front of her father. I couldn't stop myself.

When I implored Ben to work on her attitude toward me, I'd ask why he allowed Maddie to behave like such a bitch (or cunt) to me and anyone else she deemed unimportant, such as his friends. I told him I was embarrassed for him by her behavior. He insisted that he wasn't embarrassed, but he also agreed to talk to her and urge her to be more kind.

· · · · · · · · · · · ·

When Maddie planned to return to our house a couple days after my shouting match with Eli, Ben wanted me to apologize to her. He coached me on what to say and wanted to be present to hopefully help the two of us come to a truce. On the night I was to say sorry, Ben and I went together to her bedroom for my big, grand gesture. We stood in the doorway of her bedroom while she lay on her back on her bed scrolling on her phone. As I spoke my apology, she mumbled, "okay" a few times without looking away from her phone.

The main point I wanted to get across was that I had no desire to replace her mother; I just wanted to be her friend. After just a couple minutes of explaining myself, it was obvious by the annoyed tone her "okays" had taken that I'd crossed the invisible line of her tolerance for me, and I stopped talking. I turned from the doorway and walked away thinking that she was an unredeemable bitch. Ben walked away with faith that his baby girl and I had turned a corner toward a better relationship, which we had not.

Around that time, I downloaded an e-book about being a step-mother, hoping that I'd gain some insight into how to better coexist with these kids. The book's author, Wednesday Martin, a stepmother herself, had written *Stepmonster* to help people like me understand what we'd gotten ourselves into by falling in love with a man who had kids.

According to the book, the divorce rate amongst people with kids who remarry a person with kids is a whopping 70 percent. The struggle to stay married is even harder for childless women attempting to merge with a man who has children, especially if those children are girls. And wouldn't you know it, the worst time to become involved with a man who has a daughter is when the girl is between the ages of ten and sixteen. Maddie was eleven when I met Ben and currently fourteen.

The book also said that kids have an easier time accepting their mother's new mate than their father's. For some reason, they're less afraid of their parents' inability to fall in love again if the mother has a boyfriend than if the father finds himself a new companion. The context to this is that they never give up hope that their parents will remarry, not even when they grow up and move out of the house. That bit of knowledge helped explain why Ben's three kids mostly got along with Wrench Boy. It didn't seem to matter that he'd cheated with Deborah while Ben was still living in their marital house; the kids told their father that Wrench Boy was their friend.

Another disheartening fact I took from the book is the way in which the birth mother interferes with her children's relationship with the stepmom. Even though Deborah never stepped foot inside our front door, she was a constant presence in our home, and a nuisance at that. Some women overtly interfere, but others hide their evilness through such seemingly innocent tactics as constantly calling the kids while they're with their father or dropping by to bring the kids one thing or another. It's their way of making sure the kids have no reason to turn to the stepmom for guidance or help.

As an example, after Maddie got her first period, Deborah made many trips to our house to deliver a drugstore bag full of maxi pads and other supplies, along with an obligatory sugary drink from Starbucks. Maddie could've asked me for help, but she didn't have to because mommy dearest was just a phone call away and would seemingly drop whatever she was doing to run right over. Maddie would come charging down the stairs, run through the front door, return after a few seconds with a Walgreens bag and a Starbucks drink, and head back up to her room without a word.

Maddie only used maxi pads; Deborah probably thought Maddie's vagina was too fragile for an intrusive tampon. Her friends' mothers apparently didn't have the same thoughts; those girls had no trouble coming to me and asking for a tampon when they came over for a swim or sleepover. Maddie, though, only went to her mother for help.

After we moved into our jointly owned house, I noticed Maddie kept her maxi pads next to her toilet in the same white plastic bag her mother delivered them in. The way her bathroom was set up, the toilet was in a separate room from the vanity, which allowed for a person to use the double sinks while someone else could be doing their business in the little toilet room. It was a nice idea, but also inconvenient if you had your period and couldn't reach your stash of pads in the vanity.

I suggested to Ben that we buy an over-the-toilet storage unit to make Maddie's life easier and provide some privacy for her feminine hygiene products. He and I went shopping for the unit that would allow her to store her pads within easy reach. When Maddie returned to our house on her next scheduled visit, Ben showed her the addition to her bathroom and told her it had been my idea to provide her this convenience. My efforts did nothing to make her see me as someone who cared about her wellbeing and to whom she could turn to for support.

Deborah was a licensed family therapist; I had to believe she knew full well the effects of divorce on kids. She could've helped broker peace at our house—for the benefit of the kids, not for me or Ben. Instead, she was just a strange woman who I saw from a distance at volleyball games, graduation ceremonies, and musicals, and who made regular visits to our address at her daughter's request.

I don't know that her repeated visits to drop things off were an attempt to disrupt our lives, but they sure had that effect. Maddie was stubborn in her loyalty to her mom, which was never tested by me. I didn't want to be the girl's mother or cause any kind of tug-of-war between Deborah and myself; I just couldn't grasp why Maddie's loyalty meant she couldn't accept me as a friend.

Overall, I gained a lot of insight from *Stepmonster* and I was glad to have read it. But unfortunately, I didn't gain much hope that my relationship with Ben's kids would ever be anything other than shitty.

Chapter 24
Finally, Israel

Ben and I had just passed our three-year anniversary of dating and finally, I was going to meet his parents and see Israel, his country of origin. The trip was all set up, with tickets, passports, and places to stay, but there was one problem: I was having second thoughts. Truth was, I had zero desire to go with the kids. Aside from the usual difficulties—Maddie ignoring me and Eli's hypochondria and bathroom challenges, there was an extra layer of tension: I'd just had the big fight with Eli, and our truce was fragile; too much togetherness was risky. I thought it would've been better for Ben to go with just the kids and I'd stay home. I wouldn't have been offended if that's what he'd wanted to do; I had a foreboding feeling that no good was going to come of this trip.

Ben and I talked over my thoughts on Israel, including the recent conflict with Eli and how it would be a complete drag for me if Maddie did her usual and treated me like a non-person. Ben assured me that things would be fine with Eli and promised me that he'd work on Maddie while we were over there to ensure she was polite to me. Maddie was fourteen; it was beyond time she started acting like a decent human being. His mom also vowed that she'd talk to Maddie about her attitude to help bring peace to our house. I was happy to finally have recognition from outsiders, who weren't relatives or friends of mine, that Maddie's ongoing rudeness was out of line.

I still loved Ben and didn't want to give up on us. I wanted to believe him when he said he'd help with Maddie. So perhaps against my better judgement, I didn't cancel. Plus, the trip had been scheduled for months and Ben wanted me to be there, so we moved forward with our plans.

To add to my apprehension about the trip, one of my upper left molars had decided to cause problems. Shortly before our departure, it became infected and would need to be pulled. I'd already had a root canal performed twice on that tooth, and it should've been beyond dead with no possibility of further infection.

I wasn't going to travel to meet Ben's parents with one less tooth in my mouth, even if the gap wouldn't be visible when I smiled or laughed. The extraction would have to wait until after my return. In the meantime, I'd take an antibacterial medication, for the duration of our travels, to kill the infection. I already had to take my secret Zika medication daily; I'd just add this newest pill to my routine.

I had quite a bit of travel in my background; in my early twenties, I backpacked twice in Europe—once for four months and, a couple years later, for one month. When I lived in Mexico, I saw as much of the country as I could by bus. I loved road trips as much for the opportunity to pig out on Cheetos while driving, as for the sights, no matter how small, along the way. My traveling mostly came to a halt after I got married, as Leo was too cheap to spend any money on having fun. After my divorce, I took myself to Scotland, solo, to celebrate my fortieth birthday and to begin the process of catching up on my travel goals; I wanted to see the world.

Ben liked to travel and we'd talked about destinations from Hawaii to Thailand to Europe. I would've liked if these plans included just me and him, but his hope was always that his kids would tag along.

Soon after Tyler's graduation, he and Eli left to do some traveling on their own in Europe and Israel and would meet us at Ben's sister's high-rise apartment in Tel Aviv the day after our arrival. Neither boy worked or had savings, but luckily, they had parents with deep pockets who gave them money for cars, trips, and other important leisure activities that they hadn't earned or deserved. But it was sure nice that they were away, because the silence in our house leading up to the trip was golden. I loved every minute knowing that when I came home from work, it would be to a peaceful house with no kids (except Maddie during her custodial stays) and no kids' friends.

Interestingly enough, Maddie had softened toward me in the weeks leading up to the trip and it appeared as if she was making an effort to be a decent person. I started to wonder if maybe she'd turned over a new leaf. She helped me and Ben with yardwork on one occasion and was semi-talkative during an outing to Chili's. I responded by attempting to keep the conversation going, until the mean little girl I was used to reared her ugly head and I could tell it was time for me to back off. Ben witnessed the interaction and said nothing. I pretended like my feelings weren't hurt and continued the meal with my attention toward Ben and away from the girl, hopeful that this rude regression was just a glitch and she would go back to being pleasant.

Despite the fact Maddie's change in attitude toward me was new and glitchy, I was optimistic that her willingness to change would mean a decent trip to Israel. As it turned out, the softening was all an act. Once we stepped into the Las Vegas airport, Maddie's politeness evaporated. It was like a switch had been flipped; she wouldn't speak to me or even look at me. And I realized, she'd just pretended to be my friend in the weeks leading up to the trip for fear her father would follow through on his threat to leave her at home during our vacation if she was unkind to me. That threat was no longer relevant, and her dad certainly wouldn't send her home at that point.

Instead of being someone she could respectfully tolerate, I reverted back to my status as the invisible person she abhorred. She was so young and yet so cold and calculating. And Ben regressed to being the defeated dad with his tail between his legs who couldn't, or wouldn't, control the meanness of his fourteen-year-old daughter. He said nothing to her; he just looked at me with pleading eyes to put up and shut up. I couldn't. I got mad and could not get unmad.

There were a lot of moving parts to this trip, and we'd cover a lot of ground during our nearly two-week stay. Ben and his siblings had organized an excursion to a Greek island resort as a surprise birthday present for their mother. After Greece, we would fly from Tel Aviv, where his sister lived, to Eilat on the Red Sea, his hometown and where his parent still lived. From there we'd use his mother's car to drive to Jerusalem and the Dead Sea. Despite my apprehension about traveling with Ben's kids, it sounded like a fabulous trip; I was excited about all the places we'd see. I was also happy that Ben had taken the initiative to schedule everything and all I'd have to do was follow along.

This was to be an expensive trip, and the year before, I'd used the cost as an excuse to skip Israel. But Ben wanted me to meet his parents, and he wanted his mother's help in brokering some kind of peace deal between me and Maddie; so, to ensure I'd go, he paid for the airfare while we were over there. He would've paid for my ticket from Las Vegas, too, but I didn't allow it; I wanted to contribute and felt it was the right thing to do.

Most of our nights would be spent at his sister's high-rise apartment in Tel Aviv or at Ben's childhood home in Eilat, where there would be no charge for our board or meals. Ben and I pooled some cash to cover our incidental meals and expenses, which he held onto and used when necessary. I was fine with him having control of the money until he attempted to use it to buy a souvenir Maddie had requested. I told him that no money of mine would be used to buy her nice things since she was determined to be a bitch to me. He would have to pull out his credit card to reward her with purchases. Again, I received sad eyes from Ben. Why couldn't I just act happy and accept our living situation as it was?

Maddie was her usual unpleasant self, making it known to her Israeli family that she didn't like me. If ever we were all standing around in a group outside, she'd place herself in front of me with her back to me and box me out of the circle. Ben claimed not to notice it, and even after I pointed out what she was doing, he swore her actions were coincidental and not intentional.

Meanwhile, while we were in Tel Aviv, Eli had another one of his stomach episodes and needed to lie down in bed. Apparently, he'd had stomach problems all through his travels with Tyler. Tyler said they'd be having a good time socializing with fellow travelers and suddenly Eli would lay his head on the table and insist on retreating to their lodging because he was sick. The scenario repeated itself over and over and Tyler had gotten downright fed up with it.

Nobody flinched when Eli spoke of his pain; only Ben seemed worried. Ben didn't seem to mind anyone's lack of concern except for mine. He was saddened and embarrassed that I didn't show any sympathy for Eli.

Ben's disappointment with my non-existent motherliness came to a head when Tyler came down with a bellyache that same day as well. Unlike Eli's tummy problem, Tyler's was real. He'd been out late the night before with a friend from college who happened to be in Tel Aviv, and he figured he'd eaten tainted food at the bar they visited. Both boys ended up in bed late in the afternoon until the next morning.

Ben wanted to know why I didn't express any interest or care in his sons. According to him, I should've gone to the bedroom to check on them and ask if they were OK or if they needed me to "fry them an egg." I told him exactly why—one was eighteen and the other twenty-one. Eli was set to turn nineteen while we were on this trip. His boys weren't children and could handle resting until their illnesses, real or fake, passed.

A couple days after the stomachache, Eli also got bit by a cold. On the night before we were to leave for Greece, I awoke to the sound of him coughing and spitting into the toilet in the bathroom across the hall; he had graciously left the door open and lights on to make sure he was seen and heard. I didn't get up to check on him because what I heard wasn't the deep cough of a truly sick person. My sister has severe allergies and routine nasal infections and I grew up familiar with all manner of coughing sounds.

Ben and Renae ended up rushing Eli to the emergency room where, after a six-hour wait to be seen because people with real injuries and illnesses were ahead of them, they were told Eli had a cold. The trio was sent away with advice to buy over-the-counter medicine from a pharmacy. I could've given them that same recommendation and saved them time and money.

Eli, Renae, and Ben arrived back to the apartment just in time to head out to the airport for our flight to Greece. The first leg of the trip was rough on Ben because he was worn out from the late night at the ER; soon after we arrived at our resort and got to our room, he fell into a deep sleep. I had no idea where everyone else was within the resort, so I decided to head out for a walk around the town to kill time. When

I arrived back at our room after a couple hours of walking, Ben was upset because he'd had no idea where I'd gone. I was upset because I'd had no idea where everyone else was.

Most of the adults in our group, minus me, were part of a group chat on WhatsApp and were consistently updating each other on all their coming and goings. Apparently, they had decided through the WhatsApp chat to meet at the resort's beach after getting settled into their rooms, which were scattered in different sections of the property. When Ben woke up, he was able to find out where everyone else had gone through the WhatsApp chat. He was immediately annoyed with me, though, because I had seemingly disappeared.

Once off the resort property, I realized I didn't have Wi-Fi. I probably should've turned around and headed back to our room to leave some kind of note explaining my whereabouts. Instead, I chose to keep walking because I was an outsider in Ben's family anyway. Nobody had made an effort to include me, so I felt no obligation to include them in my plans either.

Shortly after I returned to our room and Ben's disappointment, we joined his family at the beach. Ben's mother thought I'd gotten lost and had been worried about me. I explained that I had no idea where anyone was and decided to go for a walk. At that point, Ben's mom added me to their family WhatsApp chat. Even if the conversation was written in Hebrew, I could translate it with Google and be up to date on everyone's whereabouts. It was such a simple solution and I was grateful to be included.

Still, because of the language barrier, I often felt left out during the trip, and my feelings were easily hurt. When the family was together, the conversation was naturally in Hebrew. A few times during the trip, we'd be at a restaurant sitting around a table with plenty of conversation going on around me in Hebrew. Since I couldn't follow along with the talk, I'd turn to my phone and an e-book or text with my family in Wisconsin to make my existence at the table a little less awkward. All at once, the entire table would stand to leave and I'd have no idea what the plan was.

The way Ben looked at me at dinner while I was on my phone, I could tell he thought I was rude for not participating in the conversation. Behind closed doors, he said that I could attempt to join in by offering up topics in English. I pointed out the number of times I'd tried to speak to his family members in English, but that after a few minutes of talking politely, the conversation couldn't evolve because their knowledge of English was limited and my knowledge of Hebrew was virtually non-existent. So, our English talk would peter out and they'd return to chatting with others in Hebrew. I also reminded him of the time I'd spent talking to Elan's girlfriend's ten-year-old son, whose English was pretty good. Just like I'd talk to the kids at David and Shuli's dinner parties while the adults spoke in Hebrew, I found a similar situation with the little boy in Israel. He was a nice kid and I didn't mind talking to him.

Aside from not talking at dinner, Ben didn't like my need for alone time, even if I was just being alone with my phone while sitting with a group. There were plenty of times during our travels when Ben's kids and his brother's three children, all of whom could've participated in the Hebrew conversation, would turn to their phones to text with friends back home or play games. But their self-isolation didn't bother him, only mine.

Meanwhile, I grew angry many times on the trip because Ben's promise to help broker peace between Maddie and me was bullshit. Nobody had the balls to tell Maddie she needed to grow up and be—at the very least—minimally civil to me. At the Dead Sea, she wanted to go to the locker room to change into her bathing suit but didn't want to go alone, and neither of her brothers would go with her. I went to the locker room, and she could have easily gone in with me, but then she would've had to acknowledge that I existed. Instead, she chose to pout. And of course, no one—not Ben, not Tyler, not Eli—told her to stop pouting and go in with me.

Rather than work on Maddie's personality flaws, it turned out that Ben and his mom were secretly working on mine. Ben would have a conversation with his mother in Hebrew, sometimes in front of me, and then later explain to me that Miriam said some aspect of my personality he questioned was acceptable. Rather than feel good that his mother was on my side, I was angered that not only was Ben breaking his promise to me by ignoring Maddie's behavior, but that he had the gall to consult his mother about *my* behavior!

Part II - Depressed & Afraid

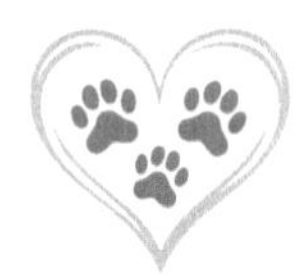

Chapter 25
The Breaking Point

There were just enough family members—and me—in our Greece travel group that we were able to each hold a Hebrew letter spelling out "Happy Birthday" in honor of Miriam. We stood in a line holding our letters and a stranger took the photo. Ben's brother had an oversized print framed and hung on the wall of Miriam's house, replacing an older family photo that included Deborah. I found it funny that the old photo contained a woman who was no longer in Ben's life, and the new photo contained a woman who might not be in his life much longer. This photo was payback for Ben taking part in my family's portrait during his first trip to Wisconsin with me.

Israel was one of the most interesting places I'd experienced and I was grateful to have gotten to see it with an Israeli. So much about the country and its history fascinated me, including walking along streets in Jerusalem that Jesus may have walked on, swimming in the Red Sea and wondering where Moses may have parted it, and floating in the waters of the Dead Sea. I'd heard about these mythical places during my Catholic school years and it was mind- blowing to see them in person.

It was also mind-blowing to travel in a country that was so news-worthy for the conflict that surrounded it; the neighboring countries desired nothing more than to remove it from existence. Ben showed me the bomb shelter in his hometown that was designated for his family and his neighbors. These shelters were ubiquitous around Eilat, and every family knew which one they were to occupy with their neighbors if a bombing were to occur. His sister's high-rise building in Tel Aviv, like all others, had one room designated as a bomb shelter. You could get no Internet signal while in that room, which happened to be the bedroom Ben and I slept in, because the walls were so thick.

There were high moments from the trip, particularly time I spent just with Ben. He and I went for walks alone while in his hometown; he told me stories from his childhood and talked about having a retirement home in Eilat. Despite the fact his daughter was an asshole to me and that he would do nothing about it, we had a lot of sex during the vacation and Ben told me repeatedly that he wasn't a quitter and we'd figure out our problems. I liked hearing those words from him and his resistance to giving up made me feel bad for doubting I could tolerate a future together.

During our stay in Eilat, Ben and I went with his brother to check out a property investment opportunity. I had $80,000 sitting in my savings account and Ben had ideas on how I could invest it . . . in Israel, where I was not a citizen, and I didn't speak the language. Signing a contract in Hebrew would've been ludicrous on my part without having one-hundred percent confidence in Ben that he wouldn't screw me over and take my investment if we were to break up, and I did not have that sense of security. I saw how he hid money from his business partner and best friend, David, and was suspicious that if there came a day that he and I parted ways, I'd never see my $80,000 again.

Ben's idea was to purchase an apartment that would be used as a short-term rental leased to tourists coming to Eilat to enjoy wind surfing and snorkeling in the Red Sea. Renters would pay the mortgage until the day we were ready to cash in and buy a house in Eilat, where we'd stay on our extended visits to Israel once we retired. It all sounded so good, but I wasn't even sure if we'd make it through the next few months back in Las Vegas.

He found the perfect apartment in a four-story building a couple miles from the water. The building was nothing spectacular and the apartment was no bigger than a standard two-car American garage. The bathroom in this apartment reminded me of what you'd see in an RV. The best word to describe everything in this apartment was small—small kitchen, small living room, small bedroom, small bathroom.

The conversation with the real estate agent started out in English, but it didn't take long before the three men turned to Hebrew. It felt weird and a tad disrespectful to not be included in the conversation when I was the buyer. I took a seat on the living room couch, which was also small, and let the men hash it out in their native language, all the while thinking to myself there was no way I would sink money into this deal. This trip had left me doubting my ability to tolerate much more nonsense from Ben and the people he loved.

• • • • • • • • • • •

The day before we'd fly out of Tel Aviv to return to the U.S., I felt on edge. Early in the trip, while we were in Greece, it had been decided that Tyler would come to live with us back home, and I was full of apprehension about it. I worried that with Tyler there, and four of them against me, I'd be even more of a stranger in my own home. What's more, Tyler was social; he liked to drink and gather people, and I feared our house was going to become party central. With Tyler's move-in and the fact that still nobody had spoken to Maddie about her behavior, my anger and paranoia reached a high. I could tell I was on the verge of the same type of explosion that had erupted on Eli a few months prior.

That night, I used my phone to check us into our flight—Ben, Maddie, and me. Tyler and Eli would travel home a day or two later. The three of us would land in New York City first for a layover, then continue on to Vegas.

My quiet stewing about the blind eye everyone had turned toward Maddie's treatment of me was at the boiling point. To protect my sanity during this long trip home, during the check-in process I changed my seat from one next to Ben and Maddie to the opposite side of the plane and further back. On the plane ride there, we'd all sat together—Maddie insisted on the aisle seat, Ben insisted on the window seat, and I got the middle, where I sat invisible. Maddie talked over and around me to her father, ignoring me altogether. I wasn't going to let that happen again. Sitting between Ben and Maddie would only add fuel to the fire that was growing inside me.

On the morning of our return flight, the three of us stood in the living room of his sister's apartment and said our goodbyes. Miriam had joined us from Eilat for the last few days of our stay in Tel Aviv. She hugged me goodbye and said I love you, which struck me as odd. I didn't feel like there was love between us; maybe a burgeoning friendship, or maybe tolerance and acceptance of each other because we both loved Ben, but not love. I said it back because I felt it was the polite thing to do.

I couldn't wait to get out of that apartment. I was ready to be done with the trip and back in my own territory. During the taxi ride to the airport, I was a little uneasy about the fight I knew was inevitable when Ben realized our seats weren't together. But then Maddie started talking in Hebrew to Ben while we waited in a long, slow-moving line at the airport to check our bags and I felt justified.

All of Ben's kids studied Hebrew at their private Jewish school and knew enough to get by. Unlike her brothers, who generally attempted to speak the language when their father or family members spoke to them in Hebrew, Maddie answered in English. However, at the airport, she spoke in Hebrew in an obvious attempt to shut me out.

Ben had made a promise to me just days earlier that when I was around, all communication between him and his kids would be in English. It was not a request I'd made; it was Ben's attempt to make me feel more included.

The promise came about after Ben grew aggravated with me for reading or going for a solo walk while he and his family communicated in Hebrew. He'd been down this road before, with the Jewish woman he'd dated within months of separating from Deborah. He'd moved her and her three adolescent kids into his house shortly after their relationship started and brought her to Israel to meet his family. Ben's version of the story was that she was a drunk who became extremely inebriated one night out at dinner with his family and needed to be carried to the car. She humiliated him, he said. But he also told me she felt left out often because everyone spoke in Hebrew but her. Thankfully I wasn't a drinker because I could've easily overindulged to keep myself busy while everyone around me talked and laughed and enjoyed their conversation immensely, which is what they did to me.

I love languages and studied Spanish and French in college. I spent eleven years married to a man who spoke to me in Spanish daily. People speaking another language other than English didn't bother me. But being roasted by Ben for not participating in conversations in Hebrew irked me.

Ben said he'd enforce an English-only rule between him, his kids, and me. But here we were at the airport and Maddie was standing there talking in Hebrew, a language I hadn't heard her speak in the three years I'd been dating her dad, knowing I didn't speak it. In front of her, I asked Ben what happened to his English-only rule. He said nothing. And I said nothing about our seating arrangement on the plane. I was just a little excited for him to see that I could be a bitch too and I wasn't going to put up with his daughter's bullshit on our travels home.

Ben and Maddie boarded the plane ahead of me. There were about 500 people waiting to find their seats and it was easy for me to let a few people slip between us. Rows of three seats lined both sides of the plane and four-seat rows took up the middle. Ben didn't notice until he sat down that I was not behind him. He and Maddie walked down the aisle on the left of the plane, and I crossed over to walk on the right side to my seat, far from that girl.

I took my seat and watched as Ben stood as best he could from his window seat and looked around for me. Our eyes met for a second and I looked away. He scooted past the person in the middle seat and his daughter, in the aisle seat, and came over to ask me why we weren't sitting together. I told him I'd purposely changed my seat the night before and would sit alone because I couldn't take him sitting by quietly while his daughter was so rude to me.

Ben looked defeated and sad as he left me and returned to his seat. He looked even more defeated when we arrived for our layover in New York and I kept my distance from him and Maddie. He came to me and asked me to sit by the two of them. I asked if he was going to allow his daughter to continue to treat me like a ghost. He again had no answer, so I maintained my distance and stewed in my anger at the continued disrespect from both of them.

After we'd landed in Las Vegas and were in the airport, Maddie passed me exiting a restroom as I entered and performed a perfect job of pretending she didn't see me, know me, or give two shits about me. And that was it—my breaking point.

I'd gone into the Israel trip hoping that things could be different with Maddie. I'd seen a glimmer of change before our trip, so I knew she was capable of it, and I'd trusted Ben when he said he'd talk to her. But that trust had been broken.

Three years. Maddie had snubbed and ignored me for three years, two of them when we were cohabitating. To be treated like this by a child for so long—as if I weren't worthy of her respect or even acknowledgment—had become more than I could take. I decided it was time for me to confront her, since nobody else had the balls to do it, and ask why she'd treated me like crap for so long.

I trudged from the restroom toward baggage claim, tired, worn down, and seeking out my nemesis. Jostling my way through the crowds, I quickly formulated in my head what I was going to say. Throngs of tourists were headed to their luggage and the start of a fabulous vacation, ready to see what Las Vegas had to offer. Maybe one of them would go home with a jackpot and plans for a better life. Maybe I was about to destroy my life and end up single with herpes by giving that little girl a much-deserved piece of my mind. It was going to be a glorious confrontation!

I got to baggage claim and my eyes locked in on her. She and Ben had already collected our bags and were waiting for me. I walked straight to her and asked pointedly, "Did you see me in the bathroom?"

"Yeah," she replied, without making any eye contact. She appeared unbothered by my question.

"Why is it, exactly, that you treat me like a ghost?" I asked her, my voice rising. "Your behavior toward me and other people—your father's friends—is *embarrassing* for your dad." I knew he wasn't embarrassed though. I wanted her to think he was.

I didn't stop there. She was disrespectful and childish, I told her. She tried to get her way by pouting like a baby.

She rushed in horror to a nearby pillar and pinned her body to it, face first, as if she'd been placed in timeout. Head hung low, she began to cry.

I could've stopped there, but I was on a roll; there was no stopping me. "You need to explain *why* it's alright for you to be so awful to me—to have been so awful for the *past three years!*"

During the entirety of my tirade, Ben had stood by and implored me to stop in both English and Hebrew. The command, "Dai!" was one of the few Hebrew words I'd picked up in my three years with Ben. It meant stop. I couldn't.

Every ounce of hatred I felt for her spewed out of my mouth. It wasn't just aimed at her, but at her father and mother, as well, for failing to rein in this kid's horrible attitude. I was glad Ben heard what I had to say. All of it was meant for him as much as for her.

Maddie had no response to the verbal spears I threw at her, uttering not a word in her own defense nor in anger against me.

My rant was over, and I stood there looking at the two of them. At that point, it made no difference who was right and who was wrong in the conflict I'd brought to light. In remaining quiet and weeping, Maddie had won this fight that I'd started.

Finally, I took out my phone and ordered an Uber for them. My Cadillac had been parked in long-term economy parking during our vacation, and I refused to allow Maddie to ride home in it. It was pointless, though, as Ben wouldn't have allowed her to get in the car with me anyway. Maddie called her mom, who dropped everything to come to the rescue and usher Maddie off to the safety of her house. I cancelled the Uber.

As I drove myself and Ben back to our house, we fought for the entire thirty-minute ride. I don't remember what he said in defense of his daughter, but it was enough to take my anger to a new level. From the driver's seat, I flung my right forearm to connect with his chest and screamed at him to just shut the fuck up!

Ben and I were done. I was free.

Chapter 26
Ten Percent

When Ben and I broke up, it was one-hundred percent mutual. I didn't have a lot of stuff because most of my things had been sold in garage sales by my first renter. I boxed up what I had and left it in the garage and took myself and my suitcases to Nancy's house.

The first couple days at Nancy's were filled with lots of chatter: talking to Nancy, calling my sister and my mom, and breaking down the drama. To my nearest and dearest, I recounted the whole story: how I'd finally drawn a line in the sand and how good it felt. My friends and family couldn't understand why I hadn't left Ben long before and weren't surprised that it had ended.

By the third day, things had calmed down a little. I'd talked everything out at length, for hours and hours, and then I was left with my thoughts. For three years I'd put off dealing with my herpes diagnosis. I'd put it on the back burner so that I didn't need to face the shame and embarrassment. I was content knowing that both Ben and I had it, and knowing that it didn't bother Ben, who would remind me, reassuringly, that it wasn't going to kill us.

But now, without Ben, herpes slapped me in the face. I was terrified of the consequences of my anger, which had left me alone, without a partner. I had become Jenny, the roommate with herpes from years ago. The one that my sister and I feared would give us her disgusting virus if we shared the same toilet or bar of soap. Now I would find out what it would be like to be single and undatable.

I thought about going on dates, possibly meeting someone I liked, and wanting to be intimate with that person. I would need to tell him about the virus. I pictured awkward silences, awkward expressions, maybe him heading for the door. *Oh, the humiliation.* I'd be left with a solitary life as a hideous leper. A life of loneliness. It would be too much to take.

I didn't want to be lonely. I wanted a partner to do things with. I wanted to go out to dinner and go to the movies and go for walks with this person. So that left me with one choice: I had to get back together with Ben.

•••••••••••

As sure as I felt about the breakup initially, I'd thought in the back of my mind that my move-out would be temporary because I assumed Ben's fear of being single with herpes was as severe as mine. I assumed the breakup, while providing me with a nice respite from living with his kids, would give him the scare he needed to realize I was serious about wanting major change in our life. I wanted respect from the kids and consequences if they were to continue being jerks, and to get me back, he'd need to give me what I wanted. But as it turned out, Ben wasn't interested in giving his kids consequences; the only consequence I got from moving out was an order from Ben to stay out.

While I was gone, Ben had been talking to *a lot of* people and getting *a lot of* advice about what he should do about me, even from people he barely knew. Apparently, Moshe told him, "Get rid of her," after finding out that I often referred to Maddie as a bitch and a cunt. *Who the heck was Moshe?* We'd met him and his wife on one occasion when they happened to be at a Hanukkah dinner we attended our first year as a couple. Ben hadn't mentioned Moshe since. But lo and behold, Moshe's opinion turned out to have as much value as those who were closer to him, who'd also advised him to dump me.

I knew family and friends were telling Ben to break things off with me, because he'd inform me of this when I called and texted him. I contacted him frequently in the weeks immediately after our breakup out of fear that he'd forget about me and move on. But rather than remind Ben what a great person I was, my frequent reach-outs served as an annoyance that gave him the chance to tell me what his friends and family thought about me and how wrong I was for him and his kids.

Ben said he'd had a nice dinner out with Moshe and his wife and David and Shuli, which took place within days after our return from Israel. The dinner couldn't have happened if I were around because of my dislike, Ben said, for his business partner and the partner's wife. It didn't matter that he didn't like them either. Both couples bent sympathetic ears to Ben's version of the story and concluded that there was no going back with me. His kids came first, they said.

His mom, the woman who'd said she loved me just a week earlier, had lost her loving feeling. She told Ben all the things she'd observed during our stay in Israel that were wrong with me, which included not being enough like Elan's girlfriend, Ina, who pitched in and folded clothes she saw sitting in a clothes basket at Miriam's house. The clothes belonged to Ben, me, and his kids, and had been washed by Miriam because only she was allowed to touch the ancient, stacked washer and dryer that her appliance repairman husband kept working. She told Ben that Ina had no idea who the clothes belonged to but naturally lent a hand and folded the clothes while I sat in the living room, in sight of the clothes basket, and read a book on my phone.

I asked Ben if he'd told his mom how I'd swept the floor one morning after she and her husband had gone to work. His and Elan's kids had made a mess all over the tiled living room floor the night before, cracking and eating peanuts. He said no, he hadn't mentioned that fact to his mom. I asked if he'd reminded her of my natural tendency to help clear the table after meals. I also offered to wash the dishes, but Miriam insisted on washing them herself. He hadn't reminded her of my efforts to pitch in for dish duty either.

· · · ● · ● · · ·

When I think back to those first few months after the breakup, I really don't know how I survived it. On top of not being able to sleep, I could feel my heart beating in my stomach when I lay down for the night. I had an infected molar I had to have pulled. I had anxiety and depression and couldn't eat. I had chronic diarrhea caused from being on antibiotics for the infected tooth, or possibly from some bacteria I picked up while traveling. And I was taking Xarelto for a deep vein thrombosis blood clot that developed in my left calf during the flight home, as well as anti-depressants for the sad state of my mental condition. I'd never experienced so much bad luck in all my life. I asked myself continually what I'd done to deserve this bad karma.

Despite all the negativity Ben was hearing about me from his loved ones and Moshe, he agreed to give me a second chance. I went over to the house one evening for dinner with Ben, Eli, Victoria, Tyler, and two girls Tyler had invited to spend the weekend. He'd met one of the girls while traveling in Israel, and she happened to be from southern California. She spent her nights in Tyler's room and the friend stayed in Maddie's. Tyler had taken over the room that had been Eli's and Eli had moved upstairs to the room that had been designated as Tyler's. I couldn't say a word about all the kids in the house or the sex going on in Tyler's room because I knew I was walking on eggshells with these people.

Ben and I also had sex that night. I was ready to move all my stuff back into the house from the garage, but Ben said no. He wasn't sure if Maddie would accept me and I had to be fine with the fact that I wasn't welcome in my house if Maddie rejected me.

A day or two later, it was Ben's forty-sixth birthday. He spent it in the pool with his kids. I wasn't invited because Maddie would be there.

During that pool time, he had a talk with Maddie about me. She told him I wasn't a bad person and her feelings toward me weren't hate. She just didn't feel we had "chemistry." That explanation did nothing to account for why she'd chosen to be so mean and intolerant of me. But it also gave me a little hope that maybe the girl and I could mend our relationship and start over.

I suggested he and I meet with Maddie and her mother at a Starbucks to have a conversation that could be the start of peace between us, which would mean Ben and I could get back together, and I could move back into my home. Ben saw things differently. He said there was no reason for a meeting between me and Maddie because he felt he and I had, at best, a 10 percent chance of getting back together.

"You weren't missed," he told me about my absence at his birthday pool party with his kids. He said I would've ruined the good time they had if I'd been there.

Soon after, in my rejected misery, I attempted to win over Eli, Tyler, and Miriam. If they only knew that Ben was the love of my life, they would surely help in my efforts to get Ben back. I didn't know how I would deal with the boys on a day-to-day basis if my attempt to reconcile was successful, but I now felt the fear of being single with herpes and I was more worried about my future than their disrespect. Why couldn't I have swallowed my pride and come to this conclusion earlier!

I texted Eli and Tyler and messaged Miriam through WhatsApp to tell them how wrong I'd been, how sorry I was for hurting Maddie, and how much I loved Ben. Only Tyler replied. His response was sweet and kind, and he wished me luck.

My friends and family were scared for me in the initial months after the breakup. I got the tooth pulled and the severe diarrhea was replaced with occasional diarrhea caused by anxiety. A prescription for blood thinners took care of the deep vein thrombosis. My physical health was somewhat better, yet my mental health showed no signs of improving. For months after the breakup, I was quick to get angry and lash out. I cried at the drop of a hat no matter where I was—at work, at a restaurant, at the movies. When the reality of being single with herpes sank in, the tears came and there was no stopping them.

If there were a silver lining to my severe depression, it was weight loss. I got skinny...oh so beautifully skinny! I lost twenty pounds without effort. The only other time I'd been able to drop that amount of weight was in my late twenties when I exercised two times per day and survived on protein shakes. I'd failed to maintain that protein-shake-induced weight loss for more than a few months because I was tired of starving. Before long, I had returned to my homeostasis weight.

This time around, the pounds came off not from effort but from the shattered state of my head and anxious condition of my stomach. I wasn't hungry and I continued to exercise. I'd take two fitness classes in a row to kill time and keep my mind occupied. Coworkers and people at my fitness center noticed I'd slimmed down and commended me on how good I looked. I took a bathroom mirror selfie to refer to if I ever wanted to remember what I looked like at my best physically (and worst mentally).

My loved ones couldn't understand why I wasn't excited to be out of the situation with Ben and the kids who had no love for me. They told me to move on and said I should be excited for the next chapter of my life and the chance to find a better man, who they were sure was waiting around every corner. What I couldn't tell them was that I was scared shitless *because I had herpes and no decent man was going to want me!*

Sleeplessness was the new norm for me. As I lay in the full-size bed in the bedroom that used to belong to one of my friend Nancy's three adult sons, my head pounded. I felt my heart beating in my stomach, and I cried and cried and cried. I could find no sleep; only worry, misery, and tears. Ben and his three kids were no doubt sleeping like babies in the beautiful five-bedroom house he and I had bought together about a year earlier, thanks to my credit.

· · · · ●· ● · · · ·

Herpes isn't the Zika virus. It doesn't shrink babies' heads. It's not a virus from China or the Middle East that causes severe respiratory illness and kills many of the people it infects. Herpes won't kill you; it causes only minor skin irritation occasionally. In my case, I had only one outbreak, the original. Despite all this, the virus killed my confidence and self-esteem. I was destined to be alone, I thought, unless I could reel Ben back in.

Self-respect was a thing of the past as I called and texted Ben incessantly to try and convince him that we needed to give things another go. I'd learned my lesson, I said, and I saw how being intolerant of his kids had caused problems. I would stop being the problem, I told him. If he'd just take me back, he would see that I had changed.

It didn't matter anyway. He'd met someone else before our trip to Israel and he wanted to date her. The new girl knew all about me, he said. He showed her photos from our Israel trip and she looked through my Facebook page. He wouldn't tell me anything about her except that she was a friend of one of his clients. He said he'd be embarrassed to take me back.

I was devastated.

Chapter 27

My Apartment, Part II

My apartment was on the first floor of a two-story building within a complex consisting of approximately thirty other buildings identical to the one I was living in. Each building housed eight apartments, with four on each floor. The complex was old by Vegas standards, having been built about thirty years earlier. To compete with the new shiny, high-end complexes popping up all over the Las Vegas Valley, all the apartments, including the one I rented, had been updated with stainless steel appliances, new paint, and new carpet.

My complex was about a quarter of a mile from my office. The fantasy I'd concocted several months earlier had come to fruition; I was now master of my domain, within walking distance from work. I was at the top of my totem pole. There were no negative and hateful kids to contend with in my space. Yet I was miserable—I hated it.

Aside from feeling lonely in my rental, it reminded me too much of my rental apartment in California, when I was young and still figuring out life. And now I had regressed back to being a renter and I felt lower than a loser.

The complex couldn't demand the same outrageous rents as the nearby, newer complexes with gourmet kitchens and community Zen gardens, so it fit my budget. I only needed a place to stay for a while, until I figured out what I was going to do with my life now that I couldn't return to my home and was single with herpes. I didn't need a high-end kitchen or meditation space in a communal area to help in my decision-making.

I'd stayed with Nancy for a month before moving out on my own. She was willing to rent me the bedroom I'd been using for $500 per month, utilities included, which was an awesome deal that I nonetheless couldn't accept. I needed to be on my own. I preferred to pay $1200 monthly for a two-bedroom apartment rather than be my friend's tenant.

I told myself, as well as the people who thought I shouldn't pass up the great deal Nancy offered, that renting a bedroom was regressing to my younger college years and I was too old to step backwards. But really, Nancy's house made me sad. There were too many memories within those walls of her dead husband, who had died from cancer a couple years earlier, and her three sons. Although she was a good friend to me and showed me great kindness in my time of need, I found her house depressing and I wanted out.

Ben was in the process of refinancing our house to get my name off the mortgage and title and wanted me to move the rest of my things out of the garage as soon as possible. While I didn't have much stuff, I had too much to store at Nancy's place and I would've had to hire movers to take it to storage. I thought it was a better idea to move my belongings and myself to an apartment and wait it out until I was ready to buy a house.

If I could've afforded the mortgage and maintenance on the home I owned with Ben, I would've fought to push out him and his spawn.

But I didn't have the financial means for that place, and although Ben did, he'd lied on his income taxes for years and, at least on paper, didn't have the income required to afford our house either. His tax guy had already prepared and filed amended tax returns that showed a better income, which would allow Ben to refinance. We were in a waiting game, hoping the IRS would quickly approve the amended return and free Ben to refinance, which would free me to buy a house for myself.

I had the money already for a nice down payment, and I'd have even more after Ben bought me out, once his refi was completed. I offered to sign off my name on the title in exchange for a $50,000 buyout. Forty thousand of that amount would be the return of my down payment and $10,000 would be just a little equity I felt I deserved. I had paid for the solar water heater for the pool, the tub in our master bathroom, and a few other improvements here and there. I took into consideration that my contribution toward updating our house was minimal compared to what Ben had invested, as well as the fact he'd put $12,000 down on my Cadillac, which was staying with me as my only means of transportation. I could've asked for more than fifty grand and, based on the expression on Ben's face and his quickness to accept my offer, he thought I was going to.

· · · · ●· ●· · · ·

My six-month-leased apartment was located on the corner of Fort Apache Road and Diablo Drive and was subjected to non-stop traffic noise. The racket from four lanes of passing cars, trucks, and city buses on Fort Apache was at full throttle when I went to bed and got up in the morning. I kept my TV on all night to help drown out the sound of the traffic as well as to ease my loneliness. Somehow the voices from the TV helped me feel a little less alone, and less loser-like.

Fort Apache's noise wasn't as bad as the sound from the busy highway that blanketed the one-bedroom apartment Leo and I had rented when we first married and lived in the San Francisco Bay area. We stayed in that space for two and a half years and grew so used to the loud noise of Highway 101 traffic that one night we were awoken by the sound of silence. Cops had stopped the late-night traffic going toward San Francisco, and in the opposite direction toward San Jose, to allow a crew to complete dangerous maintenance on power lines that involved the delivery of new wire from a helicopter. The silence emanating from that highway was deafening and caused us both to wake up and investigate what in the world was going on.

Leo and I had rented another one-bedroom apartment, when we first moved to Vegas, until we were able to buy a house, which also happened to be six months. I was twenty-nine and had been a home-owner ever since.

• • • ● • ● • • • •

Even though Ben said we had only a 10 percent chance of getting back together, I held out hope that he'd have some interest in the direction my life was going and that he'd visit me in my apartment. I thought maybe it would happen when it came time for the movers to pick up my things from his garage; perhaps he'd care enough to follow them back to my apartment and would help me unpack.

However, when the day came, Ben said he was busy with work and wanted me to meet the movers and direct them to the garage. Through tears I refused. His three kids were at his house and the humiliation of them seeing me move out was too much. I didn't want to give them the chance to gloat, knowing they had won. My tears also won, and Ben found the time to meet the movers. However, he didn't follow them to my apartment to see where I was living or help arrange my things.

Despite his supervision, the movers managed to grab one big item that belonged to him and deliver it to me. It was a rather large box containing outdoor furniture—two swivel chairs and a little table. I texted him that I'd bring his box back and at the same time pick up my coffee maker and my toiletries. His response was that he'd check with the kids to see if they wanted the coffee maker. If they didn't want it, I was free to take it. He failed to realize it had been a gift from him to me and I wasn't leaving without it. Luckily the kids didn't want it, and I didn't have to fight over a stupid little appliance.

The next weekend, when Eli and Maddie would be with their mother, Nancy helped me load Ben's furniture box into my Cadillac and accompanied me on the drive up to my old house. We took the box from my car and placed it in Ben's driveway. Nancy waited in the car while I went to the door and rang the doorbell. Ben acted happy to see me and followed me into the kitchen where my coffee pot waited for me. On the way, I passed by Tyler in the living room lying on the couch. The volume on the TV was rather loud as father and son had been in the middle of watching tennis.

"Hi Tyler," I said in a friendly manner. He was looking at his phone and I don't think he would've acknowledged me if I hadn't acknowledged him first. I had no doubt Tyler probably expected some kind of lunacy from me on this visit and was likely keeping his head down to avoid confrontation with a psychotic, scorned woman.

He looked up from his phone and said "Hi Dawn" politely and with friendliness.

He asked me how I was doing and we exchanged a few nice words. All the while Ben's head swiveled back and forth between us as if he were shocked by the kindness passing between me and his boy.

I grabbed the coffee maker and headed upstairs to get my toiletries while Ben waited at the bottom of the stairs. With my things, I exited the front door with the expectation that Ben would close the door behind me, officially ending this interaction. Instead, he tailed me outside to the car where Nancy was waiting and exchanged pleasantries of his own with her through the passenger side window. As I made my way to get in the car, he attempted to hug me and kiss me on the lips. I pulled away before his lips met mine and quickly got into the car. The motherfucker was already dating someone else!

On the drive back to my apartment, Nancy listened politely as I boasted how proud I was of myself for not letting him kiss me. I felt triumphant in my dismissal of him. But I also had thoughts I kept to myself because I didn't want to admit to my friend how that little show of self-respect on my part made me hopeful that Ben would have a change of heart.

He got to see how skinny I was and what he was missing. He'd told me our chances of getting back together were 10 percent, but maybe now that he'd experienced me acting level-headed with his son, and I'd done zero groveling, with no tears streaming down my face, just maybe my value in his eyes went up a bit. Maybe he would start to fear losing me if he didn't change his tune pretty quickly.

Of course, my appearance and sanity did nothing to change his mind.

Chapter 28
Coming Clean

y friends and family heard all my tales of woe on repeat. Some, like Nancy, politely listened. Others, like my sister and brother, who were in Vegas for a long-planned visit and road trip, grew tired of it. I'd bombarded them with stories of how I'd been wronged and the ways in which my relationship with Ben was fixable. It only took a couple days after arriving in Vegas for them to reach their limit and implore me to "just get over it!"

My sister reminded me of the ways in which Ben controlled me with examples she'd witnessed on his visits with me to Wisconsin. My brother told me he never liked Ben and couldn't understand what my attraction was to that scrawny, funny-looking Israeli. I felt that if they knew that Ben had given me herpes, they would understand why I was such a basket case and why I wanted him back at all costs. They would understand why my anxiety caused me to sneak off and call Ben to tell him about the events of our trip. If Ben answered and I got the chance to talk to him instead of his voicemail, I would beg him for another chance, which would cause him to become angry with me and hang up. The result of the interaction would be another downward spiral of extreme emotion and tears that angered and annoyed my siblings. I'd been the sister that took risks and traveled the world in my younger days; I was supposed to be fun and adventurous, not teary and stuck in the past, distraught over losing a man they didn't even like and weren't sad to see gone.

I knew the people close to me feared for my mental condition, and I felt that sharing my secret would make them understand why I'd become a skinny lunatic who was obsessed with a man who no longer wanted me. I came close so many times to admitting to whoever I happened to be talking to about Ben, which was pretty much anyone who would listen to me, the horrible injustice of him giving me this incurable virus, then allowing his kids to mistreat me, and now setting me free to fend for myself with a plague that made me scary in the eyes of so many people. I would consider who the person was, and what I expected his or her response to be—disgust or sympathy—and then back away because the unknown was too much.

Fear of being a subject of gossip consumed me, and I imagined that, if I divulged my secret to one person, that person would tell another, who would tell another, until finally I would walk a gauntlet of people who knew I was dirty and would look at me with disgust at work and in my personal life. I may have gotten sympathy from some people in the gauntlet, but I was sure most would have shame on their minds as they judged me for having sex and getting what I deserved. No one would invite me to their homes for fear I'd use their toilet and infect their whole family.

I felt the need to confide in someone other than my new therapist, a sixty-something-year-old man named Dan I'd found through my work's counseling services. My first three sessions with Dan were paid for by the state of Nevada as an employee benefit, and I'd been paying sixty bucks an hour to see him twice a week after. According to Dan, lots of people had herpes and plenty of them made their way through his office for therapy for one reason or another—sometimes it wasn't even for the herpes. Their HSV2 status was secondary to the main reason for their search to feel better through therapy.

I knew statistically that Dan's assertion was true. One out of every four to six people carries the herpes virus in their genitals, and up to 90 percent also carry it in their mouth. The mouth version is easily transmittable to the genitals. But where were these people? If, as Dan asserted, herpes was so common and I had nothing to be ashamed of, why was it I knew nobody else with the genital version of the virus, other than Jenny from so many years ago? There were obviously tons of people living in the shadows and they obviously had good reason to keep their mouths shut about their positive status despite the fact they were among plenty of company. The stigma was clearly too great to overcome.

In fact, I was so embarrassed that I'd divulged my secret to my coworker, Jerry, shortly after my one and only outbreak, that I'd purposely distanced myself from him due to my shame. I felt like any interaction with Jerry, no matter how fleeting and passive, would lead him to think, "Oh, here's this stupid woman again. What a shame she ruined herself with herpes."

I had no reason to think that about Jerry. As far as I knew, he hadn't even divulged my secret to his wife. It wasn't until after the breakup that I reached out to him again and I explained that my distance had been due to embarrassment. After that admission, I often ended up crying in his office because he knew the root cause of my stress and I could talk more in depth about the goings-on in my new life post-Ben.

Jerry was a great listener with a sympathetic ear, but he was busy with work and his family, which had grown to four small children under the age of seven. It was unfair for me to burden him as the sole keeper of my secret. He never told me to go away and the look on his face when he saw me coming was always welcoming, yet I feared that too much of my sadness and misery was going to cause that facial expression to, someday soon, turn to one of, "Here comes that stupid woman again to suck up all my time and energy."

I decided it was time to come clean to someone in my inner circle of friends and family and I chose Heather. She was my testing ground for determining my acceptability as a person who carried a virus people joked about and demeaned. Maybe if sharing my secret with Heather went well, I'd open up to all in my inner circle, because the burden of carrying this shame was so heavy. I hadn't even had an outbreak since the original one in August 2015. I lived a mostly healthy lifestyle with diet and exercise, yet I felt so ashamed of my little virus.

I was curious to know if Heather, as the mother of three children, would allow me to have face time with her family, at her home, ever again once she knew of my contamination. Most importantly, I wanted to know if she invited me to her house, would she be disgusted if I were to use any of her toilets or her swimming pool? Would she run into the bathroom after me with Clorox wipes to clean the toilet seat to protect her loved ones from me?

I'd been in plenty of public bathrooms with Heather and I knew she didn't use paper toilet seat protectors because she, like me, knew those ultra-thin pieces of paper don't provide any protection from potential ickiness. Herpes is a virus that is not transmitted through contact with inanimate objects. It cannot live on a bar of soap or toilet seat. But how many people know that? It needs a human host and is passed through skin-to-skin contact. Still, once a person knows of someone's herpes status, you can't unknow it. Would she be disgusted by me even though there would be zero chance of transmission between me and her or her family?

I came clean to Heather on a shopping trip in search of furniture for my apartment. As I drove the two of us to the furniture store, I told myself to just say it. So, I opened my mouth and began to explain that the reason why I was having such a hard time moving on from the breakup was because Ben had given me herpes. And then internally and quietly, I sighed in relief. I'd done it. I owned my story and broke free of the shame. I had nothing to hide and no reason to be fearful of my condition. If Heather decided to distance herself from me due to disgust or some other emotion associated with my status, so be it.

Heather was like everyone else I knew in that from the start, she couldn't understand my attraction to Ben. I'd made the weirdest decisions during my three-year relationship with him, decisions that made my loved ones wonder what was wrong with me. I just didn't seem independent anymore. My mother said words came out of my mouth that had no backing in my Wisconsin upbringing, and she'd worried about the influence that Ben seemed to have over me. But she didn't know about the herpes and my fear.

Heather was sympathetic. During the remainder of the drive, she asked me questions about the virus, including how many outbreaks I experience on a regular basis. From what I've read online about the virus, many people experience the original outbreak and then the virus goes dormant, which was my situation to a T, and many more people carry the virus without even realizing they have it because they've never experienced an outbreak. It became clear to me in that moment that the image many people have of genital herpes is that carriers suffer one continual outbreak after another. No wonder people are scared of it; they no doubt feel people who carry it are constantly contagious.

Heather said she understood my fear, but she also didn't understand why I felt my life was over now that I was single with herpes. She assured me I'd find somebody someday, and the best part about the new guy was that he wouldn't be Ben. From that day forward, she would send me "Ben's an asshole" texts regularly, with reminders of something Ben had said or done, in an effort to help me move on. The texts didn't have the intended effect, but they made me laugh and I appreciated that.

Chapter 29

Disclosure and The Talk

O nce my sister and brother went back to Wisconsin fully annoyed with me for my behavior, I started dating fast and hard to prove my lovability to the man who said I wasn't missed. Dan, my therapist, said it was OK for me to attempt dating even though barely two months had passed since the breakup. Everyone else said no way, too soon. My friends and family were right; however, I had my therapist's approval to find somebody to occupy my time and tide me over until I was mentally strong enough to truly move on, and I went for it full force.

On my first date with Ben, he'd told me about all the relationships he'd had since he separated from his wife, and I thought he was the perfect example of my coworker John's theory about breakups. John opined that when a relationship ends, one person will try to commit to a new relationship as soon as possible to prove his or her lovability and point the finger directly at the other as the crazy one who caused the breakup. Ben did exactly that after his marriage fell apart, and I did exactly that after Ben told me to hit the bricks.

My friend from yoga, Anisa, introduced me to Coach Craig Kenneth, a psychotherapist who, with his partner, Coach Margaret, produced short YouTube videos with advice to help losers like me navigate breakups, especially if the goal was to win the ex-partner back. Their educated advice was for the person dumped to go "no contact" with the partner who did the dumping. The lack of communication causes the dumper to miss the dumpee, and eventually, after an undetermined amount of time, reach out. Doing the opposite—reaching out to remind the ex of your existence—annoys and potentially destroys your chances of getting the ex back. I'd already done everything Coach Craig Kenneth said would turn off my ex and now it was time to try his advice and leave Ben alone. Dating would be my ticket to occupy my time and thoughts so that I wouldn't obsess that Ben was going to forget me if I didn't text or call.

Anisa was like most everyone else in my circle, including Coach Kenneth and Coach Margaret, in that she believed it was too soon to date. She repeated the coaches' recommendations to take time and work on myself, volunteer at nonprofits, exercise, get my hair done, and be alone. But she and the coaches didn't know my viral secret and how scared I was for the future. I tried volunteering at a cat sanctuary and found out that cleaning litter boxes did nothing to soothe my nerves. I needed to know what lay ahead for me—rejection or acceptance—and the only way to find out was to jump on dating sites and see what happened.

The bright side of my new, post-breakup weight was that I could list my body type on any dating profile as fit and athletic, rather than average, as had been the case when my one and only previous online dating experiment led to Ben.

I had a major hurdle to overcome with my HSV2 status and I hoped my lack of body fat would help men see past the huge burden I carried.

I didn't have kids, unruly or otherwise, that any potential paramour would have to compete with for my attention, which gave me a leg up in the dating pool. I also had a good job, a good deal of money in the bank at that point, and a retirement plan that didn't include leaching off a man. However, I had a huge anchor in the form of a tiny virus holding me down and I would cry thinking about the rejection I faced.

I scoured the Internet for help on how to date with herpes, where I found plenty of information from many points of view on the topic. I was amazed to find advice from people who were herpes positive and open about their condition with friends and family. I wanted to be like them—open—and I hoped someday I'd get there. Owning my status would mean my self-esteem had risen to the point I didn't give a fuck about what others thought about me.

The online advice I found was succinct on one point: You must tell whoever you're dating about your condition before becoming sexually active or you are a shit person! This divulging of the secret is referred to as, "The Talk."

I was in the dark about whether or not Ben had had The Talk with his new woman. But if past behavior predicts future behavior, he probably hadn't told her, just like he hadn't told me. When he admitted he was dating someone else, I asked how he'd met her and if she was willing to go with him to his beloved fuck fest near Palm Springs, but I didn't ask if he'd informed her about his viral infection. I felt like the question would implicate my own fear of being single with that condition and I didn't want him to know I was scared.

During our three years as a couple, I'd kept quiet that the virus was the motivating factor keeping me in the relationship. I assumed it was his, as well. However, he was already with another woman, and I knew he moved fast when it came to sex, so I assumed he and his new love were most likely sexually active. I wanted Ben to think I was fearless regardless of my herpes status, just like he appeared to be, and the way to show my fake courage would be to latch on to a new lover as soon as possible, just as he had.

Online advice differed on the right time to come clean with a potential mate and have the talk. Some people suggested telling a date prior to first meeting to avoid wasting time. Other online advisors suggested waiting until after a date or two or three to break the potentially love-ending news. They said there was no need to share your medical history with someone unless you saw, with time, that you hoped to go further with that person. The advisors even provided sample text of what to say, including statistics on how common the infection is and how unlikely you are to spread it if taking antiviral medication, which I was.

My gynecologist suggested I stop taking antivirals after a few years had passed and I hadn't had an outbreak since the original. I said absolutely no way, no how. I planned to be a lifer on those pills. I was too scared to find out what would happen if I stopped.

Back in 2015, when I'd read all about the virus online, I'd found out that there was a dating site named Positive Singles specifically for people with STDs. I didn't think I'd ever get to the point of needing to set up a dating profile on PS, as it's affectionately known amongst the online people who were now my community, but now it was time to check it out.

The upside of PS is that you would never have to have The Talk with a potential suitor. The downside is that the dating pool on the site is small despite there being a ton of people in the world with the condition. Exposing yourself on a website in which you could be potentially outed is apparently hard for most people. And for those brave enough to create a profile, many didn't have the courage to show their face in their profile pic. I was one of those people with that fear and posted a profile pic that showed my torso from the neck down.

The consensus from online advisors was to use mainstream dating sites to have access to a larger dating pool and to disclose your status prior to becoming sexually active. With this advice in mind, in addition to my PS profile, I set up an account on match.com, the same site that led me to Ben, and on bumble.com, which seemed to be a fan favorite amongst women with herpes. And then I got to work dating.

In a short amount of time, I had my first date with a Hispanic "normal" guy. I was looking for a man similar to Ben on all the sites and was immediately attracted to anyone who was an entrepreneur. A foreign entrepreneur was even better. The Hispanic guy was a realtor and did not match the type I hoped to find, but he was quick to ask me out and unwittingly helped me practice how to disclose my HSV status and experience a reaction.

We met for coffee at a place that was convenient for him. He was new to Las Vegas and living in an apartment, which he didn't seem to mind. When I asked where he was from originally, he answered California. I knew he wasn't born in the United States because he had the slightest of accents, and my guess was that he was Mexican. From my studies to become a teacher of English as a foreign language, I knew that children could learn to speak a foreign language like a native if they were immersed in the language before the age of twelve. He must've been pretty close to twelve when he ended up in California, but not close enough. He seemed a little surprised that I even asked if he was born somewhere else, but admitted that he was, as I thought, Mexican.

As we talked about our backgrounds over our coffees, I cried as I told him the story of my relationship and breakup, about how I was steamrolled into a life that didn't quite fit me and how poorly Ben's kids treated me. He provided a very sympathetic ear and committed himself right then and there to helping me get over Ben with his time and his body. He'd had a relationship in the past that was purely a bridge to get over a past love. The woman who'd provided the stepping stones to help him move past his hurt supposedly was just in the relationship to help him move on. They were like a typical couple in that they went to dinner, hung out, hiked, and had sex. But once he felt like he'd put his past love behind him, he ended it with the bridge lady, who went quietly away. He wanted to be my bridge and I agreed to it.

Of course, I left out the part of the story that involved herpes, even though it was on the tip of my tongue. I had no idea how or if I was going to tell him. I wasn't necessarily interested in hanging out with this guy, I just wanted to know if he'd accept me.

With our coffees long gone and our new relationship seemingly set in motion, I tried to bid him adieu at the cafe's exit, but he decided to be a gentleman and walk me to my vehicle. Once we were there, he gave me a deep and penetrating goodbye kiss. It took me off guard and I know my performance was subpar. He was the first guy to kiss me since Ben, and it was weird.

We went our separate ways that evening and the next day, at about midmorning, he started texting flirty messages related to our new relationship deal. After a while of back-and-forth messaging, I decided it was time to break the news about my STD status, and to begin I asked about his. He replied that he was, without a doubt, "clean."

I typed up a text that explained my HSV2 status, how I got it, and the anti-viral medication I was taking that would make transmission of the virus from me to him unlikely. Online advice suggested keeping an upbeat tone to your messaging, whether it be in writing or face-to-face. If you present your disclosure as if you're disgusted with yourself and the virus, you would be suggesting to your potential mate that you wouldn't date someone like you, and you'd understand if he didn't want to date you either. Despite the matter-of-fact tone of my disclosure, my Mexican paramour replied with utter disgust. Not only was he adamant that our deal was off, he was also disgusted that we'd even kissed the night before.

There was no need for me to reply. I deleted his contact information and that was the end of that. I knew what kind of life lay ahead for me and it wasn't pretty. I also was certain all the online information I'd read from carriers of the virus stating that life with herpes wasn't that bad was bullshit. I needed to warn Ben.

At some point that day, I ended up on the phone with Ben and told him about my first dating experience. I informed him that he really needed to rethink our breakup because it was going to be tough for us out there in the dating world. I gave him a breakdown of my experience with online advice on how to disclose you had the virus and the response from the Mexican guy. Ben was unmoved by the warning I gave him.

I thought my warning would have the effect I desired; that he would realize, through my experience, the future that lay ahead for him, and see that we were each other's best option. And then, I predicted, even though he was already dating someone else, he'd have a change of heart and take me back. As it turned out, my fear was not shared by Ben. He was fine with the direction his life was going in and was not afraid.

Not even my mirror selfie of my body in bra and underwear could persuade Ben that I was his best option. I was skinny, yet my trim physique had zero effect on convincing Ben or a new man to take a chance on me. My life was doomed.

Chapter 30
My People

A happy hour for people with herpes was scheduled for Friday night at Blue Martini in Town Square, the same place where I'd met the Egyptian guy who'd caught my attention a few days before my first date with Ben. When I arrived, the only one there was Mike, the event's host, a rather skinny White guy in his early forties who was OK-looking. It was just the two of us for a bit, which was nice because it gave me time to calm my nerves and become acquainted with at least one person before others showed up.

The next person to arrive was Nicole, a prettyish White girl in her early thirties who was pear-shaped like me, except her torso was scrawnier than mine and her butt and hips were a tad bigger. Besides herpes and pear-shaped bodies, Nicole and I also shared first-time status with this support group. Mike, Nicole, and I had a nice time talking for quite a while before our group expanded with a few more gatherers.

I'd searched Google for a herpes support group in the Las Vegas area and was quite happy and relieved to find that one actually existed on Meetup.com. I wasn't the only one in this position and it felt good not to be alone. I was ecstatic to see that there were a few hundred members in the Meetup group, and I hoped to soon call some of them friends. I was especially anxious to talk to them and learn tricks on how to deal with the virus like a boss, unafraid and optimistic about the future.

Even though I already had an existing account on Meetup.com, I started a new one with the same email address I'd used to sign up with Positive Singles. I created that address for the specific purpose of joining PS and now I'd use it for everything herpes related. Unlike my two other email accounts I'd had for at least twenty years, which I was logged into at all times on my phone, I only logged into my "herpes email" when I was alone. I had a fear that a family member or friend would look over my shoulder and see an email from PS or the herpes Meetup on my phone screen. It didn't matter that PS already disguised their emails so that a situation like I feared wouldn't happen, or that my family was thousands of miles away in Wisconsin, and that I didn't typically answer emails while with friends. My anxiety about being outed was so strong that I had to add this extra level of secretiveness to my life.

Many of the people in the herpes Meetup group, just like many of the people on PS, hid their true identities despite being required to have a profile pic in order to join. The group was private with an innocuous name that didn't scream it was for people with herpes. You had to request permission to join and be accepted by the group administrators. Part of the admittance procedure required answering questions, such as where you lived, and confirming that you did, indeed, have herpes. You also needed to have a profile pic. Many people skirted this last requirement by using a photo that showed a close-up of their eye, a pic severely altered with a filter, an avatar, or a faraway shot that obscured their appearance.

Many others used true profile pics, including me. However, I didn't reveal my face out of bravery; I used a selfie of me and Ben hugging since he was the reason I was joining this group. I thought it wasn't fair to only expose myself when he was as guilty as me. I also secretly hoped someone in the group would see that pic, recognize him, and tell him he was on display.

I expected the herpes Meetup support group to gather in a clinical setting at a hospital or a church basement, much like you'd see support group meetings on TV shows. I imagined we'd sit on folding chairs in a circle while we ate cookies, drank coffee, shared our stories, and discussed how to move on. Instead, this group planned to meet at a bar for happy hour. It was such a normal setting, and I looked forward to seeing what the group was all about.

This gathering would be the first I attended of any type of get-to-gether through the Meetup website, and I was full of anxiety about showing up alone. But I did it. I drove myself to Town Square, parked my car and walked into the bar despite the anxiety that was trying to convince me to turn around and flee. I was proud of myself for breaking out of my comfort zone.

Ben used to complain that I wasn't social enough, but here I was proving him wrong. I wished he could see me out and about so that he'd know I was strong—even if it was an act at this time—and con-tinuing on with my life. But I was also mad at him for putting me in this situation, in which I was looking for similarly afflicted people to hang out with to cope with the direction my life had taken. This new set of circumstances gave me a churning in my stomach, and I blamed Ben and his kids. And yet, I was following through with the Meetup, looking forward to meeting people who would hopefully become my friends.

Slowly, people with herpes began to trickle into Blue Martini. Mike seemed to know most of them, except for a few newbies like me and Nicole. Eventually, about fifteen people of varying ages and from all walks of life joined the gathering. I looked closely at each and every one. No one looked dirty or worthy of carrying a virus that grossed people out and made others afraid to touch them. I wanted to know their stories and how it was that they'd come to be part of this elite group. There were Black people, White people, and a red-headed Hispanic guy who was married to a Filipina woman. That couple looked to be in their early thirties and had recently moved to Las Vegas from Victorville, a small California city known as a bathroom break stopover on the way from Las Vegas to Southern California. If those two carriers could find each other in a small city, I had hope that I, too, would have such luck with undoubtedly more options in much larger Las Vegas.

From Mike, I learned that, in addition to the Meetup group, there was also a private herpes Facebook group with more than 400 members. He said that to join, an existing member of the group needed to vouch for you, which he said he'd do for both me and Nicole. I wondered for a moment if Mike could be a love option for me. He was apparently wondering the same thing about Nicole, who he ended up dating briefly. I heard all about it through my friendship that developed with Nicole.

According to Mike, many of the members created secondary, fake Facebook accounts with fake names and altered profile pics for fear of being found out. If you used your real account, you ran the risk of someone in the group inadvertently—or blatantly—outing you, which happened to Mike within months of this first meetup.

He, like me, was recently single and dating hard, for which he'd earned a reputation as being a bit of a womanizer. He especially had a taste for women at least ten years younger than him. A middle-aged Black guy named Frank took him to task for it. If Frank had blasted Mike for his behavior within the Facebook group, at least the beef between the two would've been contained amongst 400 people. Instead, Frank committed a felony in herpes society by blasting Mike on Mike's wall, where his family and friends could see. That little stunt got Frank a lifelong ban from the group.

Mike was an administrator of the Facebook group and friends with most of the members. He actually had to befriend new members to vouch for them because new members had to be vetted. Mike used his real Facebook account, which allowed Frank, his friend, to post a rambling comment on Mike's wall about his supposed prowess with women, as well as his case of the herps.

I decided I would use my true Facebook page to join the herpes group, but to avoid a situation like Frank caused Mike, I would only accept Facebook friendship with Mike because I had to. I was already logging in and out of two Meetup accounts and I didn't want the extra work with Facebook as well. Plus, I had a hope that someday I'd be OK if the world inadvertently found out I had herpes. Still, at least for the time being, I locked down my page so that nobody could message me or post on my wall.

As my membership in the Meetup and Facebook groups became more regular, I met some nice people, guys and girls, that I'm proud to call friends. We are like superheroes in that we all have origin stories to explain how we came to have our herpes superpower. We can drink from each other's cups because, we joke, we know we all have herpes.

From these friends I learned of similar Facebook groups across the country. One in Texas has a couple thousand members in it. There are even a few national groups that host social events on an annual basis. Knowing these groups exist was comforting. Life goes on and people find a way to survive and move beyond their fears. In time, I hoped to be one of those survivors and maybe even attend one of the national events.

Chapter 31

Leo

Leo and I met for dinner at California Pizza Kitchen one warm October evening at Downtown Summerlin, the outdoor mall where I'd had my first date with Ben. At my suggestion, we sat outside on the restaurant's patio to enjoy the weather. We hadn't seen or talked to each other in more than three years, and I looked forward to catching up. I arrived first and waited outside on a bench (just as I had for Ben on our first date). I saw Leo approaching with an angry look on his face.

I was a good twenty pounds lighter than the last time we'd seen each other, and he must've noticed, but chose to remain silent on the topic. Everybody else I encountered in those days commented on my weight loss. They told me I looked good and wanted to know my secret. Rather than attribute it to diet and exercise, I admitted the cause was life changes that were hard to deal with. I would've given him the same spiel if he'd mentioned my appearance. It was a bit of a letdown that he didn't say a thing.

As for him, he looked exactly the same as the day we married at the courthouse in Redwood City, California, in 1999. His body was still slim and athletic and his hair just as dark in his forties as it was in his twenties. He was a handsome man, and I hoped to hear stories about women he'd dated since our divorce, or maybe even that he was in a relationship now. His belief that he could trust no one, including me, the woman who'd had enough faith in him to bring him to America, had always made me sad and I hoped that he had changed.

Robo texts from political candidates vying for votes in the upcoming November elections had brought us together again at this dinner. As an Independent voter, I was receiving texts from both sides. However, I'd also been getting text pleas not just meant for me, but some for Leo as well. Feeling the vibration of a text from my phone in those days was a quick jolt of dopamine that I needed to help soothe my nonstop anxiety about being alone. Looking at my phone and seeing a candidate's pitch was a severe letdown. It was even worse receiving a meaningless message meant for someone else.

Leo and I had set up our cell phone accounts together shortly after moving to Las Vegas in 2002 and our phone numbers were almost exactly the same, except that the last number for each differed. Mine was 3 and his was 1. I had a suspicion that Leo, to be a dick, had written my number down on his voter application or some other list that would be accessible to candidates. After receiving more than a few political texts asking if the candidate could rely on Leo for his vote, I'd texted him to ask why he was using my phone number for whatever political activities he had going on. To my surprise, he replied fairly quickly that he hadn't.

We exchanged a few texts back and forth that were neither gushing with excitement about reconnecting, nor angry or sad. They were rather blah and matter of fact. I told him I'd broken up with my boyfriend of three years and was living temporarily in an apartment. I asked if he wanted to meet for dinner and, to my surprise, he accepted. I suggested a time and location and he agreed to it.

Leo was unforgiving and held on to anger forever. Even the smallest slight would end up in his memory bank of reasons why I, or any other person who'd offended him, could not be trusted. Any time we fought, he would list offenses from years past to prove how horrible I was and had always been to him. I should've known that Leo was so amenable to my dinner invitation because he wanted to tell me, again, to my face, that I was a bitch.

This time he was holding a grudge for my supposed poor treatment of him after I'd allowed him to move back into our house on a six-month trial basis approximately three years after our divorce. The typical fights from our marriage evolved into roommate fights based around the same themes of, "you always do this and you never do that." We returned to our old pattern of fighting and screaming at each other until we grew silent for days on end. Rather than progress into a new relationship as friends, we regressed into the same couple we had been while married. I realized that having him as a tenant had been a huge mistake.

I asked Leo to move out before the six months were up, but he refused. I was charging him a bargain rent of $500 per month, including utilities. Perhaps it was a little hard to give up, but one would think he'd have done it for peace of mind. However, the lease said he had the right to stay in my house for six months and he wasn't leaving until the last day of his legal tenancy.

At California Pizza Kitchen, I asked our waitress for separate checks before we placed our order. I knew this Mexican man, who came from a culture in which the man was expected to pay for the woman, would not offer to cover my bill. By asking for separate checks, I made it clear that I had no expectation he would pay for me and I was not going to pay for him either. His unflinching facial expression when I made the request to the waitress told me it was the right choice on my part.

This dinner would be no different from our previous lives together as husband and wife, and later as ex-spouses living together, in that we started fighting almost immediately and would come to no meeting of the minds. He accused me of cheating on him with Ben during his six-month tenancy, to which I scoffed in his face. Although he admitted at dinner that he hoped to rekindle a relationship while roommates, he said nothing to me before moving in or after. I hadn't met Ben until a couple months after Leo moved out; my conscience was clear.

It turned out the specific reason for his anger was a text I'd sent him several months after he moved out. He'd messaged me to ask if he could stop by to visit the cats, and I replied that it wouldn't be appropriate because I had a boyfriend, which was Ben. Leo remembered the text verbatim because it was an offense and offenses stuck hard to his memory. For that, Leo said, I was a bitch.

At one point, the hostess sat two middle-aged White guys, who looked like they were there to discuss business, close to Leo and me. There wasn't enough space for us to yell at each other from across our dinner table without being overheard. The two guys glanced over at us a couple times as our whispers grew heated, and again when I started crying. I was hoping to impress Leo as a confident, skinny, single woman without an incurable STD, but I accomplished exactly the opposite.

By the time Leo had texted to ask if he could visit the cats, I'd already been diagnosed with herpes. When I sent the text denying his visitation, there was more at stake than a simple trip to see the cats. I was trying to move on and be 100 percent committed to making it work with Ben so I wouldn't have to face life alone with my condition.

Leo's anger toward me turned to sympathy after I told him, through tears, that I had contracted herpes from Ben. I was broken and Leo could tell. I told him everything that had happened during the previous three years with Ben and in the few months that had passed since our breakup. Instead of hating me, Leo's hatred turned toward Ben.

Of course, we still had more to fight about. If he'd been in the same situation as me, he said, there's no way he would've stayed with the person who gave him that life sentence. He could not have cared less if he'd have to face life alone forever. He'd rather reject the herpes spreader than stay in a relationship with someone who deceived him.

I absolutely believed that this stubborn man I'd married would have had no problem facing life alone rather than staying with his "gift giver," the term people in the herpes world call the person who gave them the virus. I tried to explain to Leo my logic for staying, which did not satisfy him one bit. I wasn't like him in that I couldn't accept being shunned forever, and Leo wouldn't accept my fear of being alone as reason enough to put up with Ben and his kids. As was always the case with us, we fought to make the other see our point of view rather than just admitting our beliefs were different and moving on to another topic.

Dinner ended and we went our separate ways outside the restaurant. We didn't hug goodbye or express any sentiment that it was good to catch up. But this parting wasn't the end of our relationship together. We walked away as friends.

After my dinner with Leo, I got the bright idea to send Ben a text letting him know that I'd shared a meal with my ex-husband. As would happen frequently while alone in my apartment, especially at night, my thoughts would be laser focused on Ben. Anxiety would get the best of me, and I'd end up texting him good night or some other unnecessary, stupid text, including my note about dining with Leo. I'd reason to myself before sending the text that I would be OK if he didn't reply. But of course, I wasn't. I would end up even more anxious if I was ignored. However, to this text about Leo, he replied that he was surprised to hear Leo and I had been in contact.

He didn't reply to my follow-up text, but I was satisfied that he'd acknowledged me, and he now knew that I was capable of being cordial to exes. There was no reason why Ben and I couldn't be cordial as well. I was content that I'd made him aware that unexpected things were happening in my life and he wasn't part of them. I hoped he feared that I would move on without him if he weren't more receptive to keeping in contact. However, that last hope was the thought of a desperate woman and nowhere near reality.

· · · ● · ● · · · ·

Not long after my dinner with Leo, I decided to make a day trip on a Saturday to Zion National Park in Utah rather than face the loneliness of my apartment. I had nothing planned for that day and my anxiety about being a lonely loser was killing me. The trip would take the whole day: four hours driving there, a few hours hiking, and then four hours back. When I got home, the day would mercifully be over, and I could hit the sack. If anyone asked me what I'd done over the weekend, I'd have this spontaneous trip to Zion to tell them about; I hadn't been just crying alone in my apartment.

I invited Leo to accompany me on my day trip. Being antisocial, I expected he'd be free and I was right. It was just like in the old days when we were married—we'd fight one day and then the next, if I were willing to give up the argument, we'd go on as if nothing had happened. This guy, whose motivation for agreeing to have dinner with me days earlier was simply to tell me that I was a bitch, was now going with me on a trip to Zion and I was glad to have his company. Leo could be maddeningly stubborn, but I felt we'd always be connected on some level.

Leo's condo was only fifteen minutes from my apartment, and also only fifteen minutes from the house I owned with Ben. We'd ended up living on the same side of Las Vegas without knowing it. After his six-month tenancy with me had ended (and not a day earlier), he'd rented an apartment for a couple years near his current condo. Regular rent increases motivated him to buy his one-bedroom home, for which he'd paid $100,000 cash. He'd also purchased an apartment with cash in his home city of Guadalajara, for which he received rental income. Being cheap was paying off well for him.

He furnished his place like a man who planned only a temporary stay. His kitchen table was a portable, six-foot foldable plastic piece meant for outdoor use, and his chairs were of the same ilk. He had a lawn chair sitting in his living room and two mountain bikes—one I'd gifted him while we lived near San Francisco, and the other he'd bought for himself after we moved to North Las Vegas. He had used the second bike a couple times on excursions with coworkers. I doubted he currently used either one and I found it odd that he still possessed them and had bothered to move them from one residence to the next. His place was not set up for guests and Leo said he liked it that way.

His bedroom was as sparsely furnished as the rest of his home, with a bed that looked like it was meant for a toddler. He said he paid almost nothing for it at Big Lots. A small flat screen TV sat on the same kind of table he used in the kitchen. Napping and watching TV were so important to him while we were married, but this arrangement didn't seem conducive to the enjoyment of either activity. Leo said he barely watched TV anymore and he slept very little due to insomnia. He spent his time on his computer learning new things, like coding, he said, to pass the time. He also claimed porn was no longer interesting to him, which I found to be a more highly suspect statement than his claims of not watching TV or sleeping much. The major character traits that bothered me while we were married had apparently disappeared from his life.

With the tour over after a few minutes, we loaded ourselves into my Cadillac. It was just like the old days when we were married; I always did the driving and Leo rode shotgun. He didn't have a driver's license for the first year or two in the United States and I ended up doing all the driving because I had to. It was a pattern we developed early in our relationship and we stuck with it.

The four-hour drive to the park and back was full of conversation as we caught up on the events going on in his life and with my family. I ended up in tears several times because I was an absolute nut job and could not control my sadness. Leo didn't berate me for that. He gently massaged the back of my neck as I drove, which is something he would do occasionally while I drove during our marital days.

He told me about his dating attempts in California and Las Vegas and about his decision to be celibate. He said there were too many single mothers to contend with who had bad credit, no money, and often gambling or substance addictions. He felt like the women he met were only interested in what he could provide them, which to him was a complete turnoff. He chose to drop out of the dating world completely and live a solitary life, which he claimed fit him perfectly; he said that he wasn't lonely.

I didn't believe that he wasn't lonely. I always had a sense about him that his stubbornness and fear of being taken advantage of wouldn't allow him to admit that he wanted companionship as much as anybody else. The fact that he was going to spend all day driving to and from Zion with me was proof of that.

While we walked a trail within Zion, Leo mentioned that he and I could "try again" as a couple. He took me by surprise since I'd already disclosed to him that I had herpes. As our walk and talk continued, I realized I had to tell him no. I explained that sex was one of our biggest issues; I wanted it and he didn't. With herpes in the mix, I told him I didn't think we could overcome our sexual issues, and he agreed, with no further discussion or protestations.

Our discussion about trying again didn't lead to a fight. We didn't have to be a couple to hang out, I said; our trip to Zion was proof of that. We could go to dinner, the movies, and other events as friends. Leo made me promise that I wouldn't freeze him out if I got a boyfriend and I said I wouldn't.

To Leo, my friend, I will be forever grateful for that offer to try again. I needed a win and that was a win and a half. I must not have been half bad if my ex-husband could overlook my condition.

Chapter 32

My House

I detested weekends and looked forward to them with anxiety and fear. If by Thursday evening I had no plans for Saturday and Sunday, my head would fill with intrusive thoughts about the good times I was sure everybody else was enjoying, especially Ben, while I was the only outcast with no dinner plans or happy hours to attend. Those thoughts would wander around my head, upset my stomach, and keep me awake into the night.

I attempted to push through my anxiety and fear by forcing myself to spend time alone in my apartment until I was OK with it. Surely, if I rekindled my painting passion, the next six months of my lease would be tolerable inside this rented space. After my divorce from Leo, I would paint for hours and was grateful for the hobby that occupied so much of my time while I healed from my failed marriage. This go-round with a breakup was different. Painting required lots of time alone and being alone was the thing I feared most.

I set up my painting desk in the living room of my apartment with the intent of healing myself once again and returning to the person I'd been before Ben and herpes disrupted my life. The desk was the same cheap press-board piece of furniture from Walmart that had made its way from my North Las Vegas home to Ben's house in the north, to our joint home, and now my stupid rented space. The right side of the desk had come loose during the latest move and I used black duct tape to hold it together. I set up my paints and brushes in their usual spots on the desk, paints to the left and brushes to the right, and then I got busy avoiding painting.

I used to bitch at Ben for keeping me away from painting to accommodate his need to always be together, busy doing anything and nothing, but now there seemed to be no way to make myself get back into my craft. I decided the problem was the living space I hated so much. Residing in an apartment made me sad and, therefore, my abode was holding me back from healing. My solution was obvious: I needed to buy a house as soon as possible. Once I was in my own home, I believed I'd feel more comfortable, less like a loser, and would return to my old self.

Nancy said that common advice after a trauma is to wait at least a year before making a life-altering decision like moving or buying a house. As if waiting 365 days would somehow help ensure I didn't commit to a knee-jerk change I'd later regret! The housing market was soaring and there was a common belief that a crash was coming any day. I didn't care and I wasn't scared. The first house I ever owned, the one Leo and I bought in North Las Vegas, lost almost half its value in the Great Recession. I'd waited it out and had a hefty amount of money in my savings account because of it. I was laser-beam focused on getting a house and no amount of doubt placed in my mind from coworkers, family, or friends about buying a house in a seller's market could dissuade me.

However, there were two very real obstacles to homeownership and healing. The first obstacle was the fact that I was only a month into my six-month apartment lease and would have to pay to get out of it. The other was that I wasn't released from my mortgage yet with Ben.

The likelihood that my bank would approve me for a second mortgage while still under the thumb of my first was unlikely.

Solving the first dilemma was easy. When I make up my mind on something that previously caused me indecisiveness, I ask myself if I'd think about the decision on my deathbed and regret it. Would I look back on my life and feel stupid for paying a couple thousand dollars to break my lease? I had $80,000 in the bank and would have another $50,000 once Ben refinanced. The answer to my deathbed question was a resounding no. This same way of thinking gets me in trouble when it comes to binging on candy or cake. When I'm a dying old lady, I just don't think I'm going to regret binging M&Ms, Snickers, and cake on occasion – unless I ended up fat. And I didn't think I'd regret spending the money to break my lease either.

I wanted a home in the $300,000 range, which would likely get me around 2,000 square feet. I wanted enough backyard that I'd need to invest time in improving and maintaining it. The thing I liked most about my house with Ben had been the backyard, with its mature olive and fruit trees. I hoped my new place, even though it would be much smaller, would provide me satisfaction in the backyard as well.

Fortunately, Ben thought he'd be able to refinance the house soon. He believed that the IRS was on the verge of approving his amended tax return and with that approval, his Israeli loan officer—the same one who'd come up with the idea of using me as the primary on a joint loan with Ben—would push his refinance through.

Ben had shown a slight interest in my search for a new house, and I took advantage of that interest by reaching out with occasional phone calls and texts, being careful not to be too persistent or overdoing it. He said he'd offer his construction crew to help—at cost—with any remodeling work I needed when I found my house. He'd offered the same deal to David, his supposed best friend and business partner, and still managed to eke out a profit for himself, and I knew I'd be no different. I was just happy that he was receptive to my attempts at communication and began to believe maybe we'd have a chance at reconciliation if I could control my emotions and wait patiently for him to finish with the woman he was currently seeing.

I reasoned it was good that he was dating someone else, so he had a comparison between me and her, and ultimately, he would see I was the better choice. This belief led me to concentrate my search for a new place in the area around where Ben and I co-owned our home. I also looked around in neighborhoods closer to work and further in the opposite direction just in case the perfect house popped up; however, the houses closer to Ben drew my attention the most. If I lived near him, dating in the future would be easy geographically; I'd be just down the road. The plan I devised while we previously lived together—to live apart so he could parent his way in his house with his kids—would function. I'd be right. He'd see.

But of course, those were just the thoughts of a crazy person. In October, while my house hunt was in full swing and his amended tax return was yet to be accepted, Ben told me to quit calling and texting; his new girlfriend didn't like it.

I was on my way to take a Pilates class and I called Ben to say hello and tell him about the latest goings on in my house hunt. He had been receptive to me prior, and I was totally unprepared for him to drop the hammer on me in that way. There was no convincing him that we could remain chatty friends despite the fact he was seeing someone else. Every time I called, my face popped up on his phone caller ID and he didn't want his girlfriend to experience any distress if she happened to be around when I reached out. The solution was simple I said, remove my photo and don't tell her that he and I talk. His solution was easier – he told me to quit calling.

After the phone call, I parked my car in front of my yoga and Pilates studio and strengthened myself to go inside and have a workout. Surely this anger, disappointment, and sadness I felt would work its way out while I lifted weights and performed jumping jacks in a class of thirty people. I made it five minutes into the start of class when I felt an overwhelming need to flee. I motioned to the instructor by patting my stomach that I didn't feel well. She could probably see the anguish on my face and nodded that she understood. I packed up my mat, towel, and hand weights and left the room while the instructor's music blared and she continued to call out moves for the class to follow. I barely made it to the car before I broke down in tears.

I sat in my car in the parking lot and called my friend Mark. We'd still been meeting for lunch about once a week and he was well aware of my fragile mental state. During our lunches, I'd often end up in tears as I forced Mark to listen to the injustices forced upon me by Ben and his decision to throw me to the curb rather than make his children be nice to me. My grief was so severe that Mark worried I "wasn't going to make it." I was never suicidal, but my depression was more severe than anything I'd ever experienced, and I also wondered how I was going to come out of it. Ben's decision to stop communicating with me was another blow that ramped up my depression a notch.

It had been Mark's habit to joke about the two of us dating even while I was with Ben and he was with his girlfriend Sandy. It was harmless joking about two friends attempting to make a go of a relationship if nobody else wanted us. At least on my part, the playful banter was harmless because I didn't see any hope for us in the future. Aside from the fact that he was a compulsive dater, we lived completely different lifestyles. He liked to hang out in casino bars and drink and gamble and, although he had a room in his house dedicated to exercise equipment, he didn't exercise. He also had four stents inserted in his heart due to a heart attack he'd had years earlier. He had twelve years on me and if we got together, I thought I'd probably end up as his caretaker.

He said the characteristic he liked most about me was that I was the only woman who could make him laugh. Maybe it was true that he found my sense of humor attractive, but he also commented about visualizing himself with a younger woman. He said he would enjoy the looks on his friends' faces when he showed up at events with me on his arm while they showed up with their more age-appropriate wives. To sweeten the pot, he also joked that marrying him could make me a wealthy widow after his death. I would inherit his primary home, three or four rental properties, and the money he had in the bank.

Based on his own admissions, Mark had been with a lot of women. He told me story after story about his conquests. Knowing his sexual past, I would comment about the risk to his penis of contracting an STD. I just couldn't understand how I had an incurable STD while men like Mark, with a litany of past conquests, were disease-free, as Mark claimed to be. I wondered if he secretly had my disease or if he was one of the silent majority of HSV carriers who had no idea the virus was unknowingly harbored inside their genitals. I saw Mark as a symbol of the world's unfairness that I would have herpes and he didn't.

Every time Mark joked about us dating, I couldn't help but silently question if his joking would continue if he knew I was tainted. He didn't seem to care if the women he chose had good jobs or credit. It was a visual he seemed to be after, and I seemed to fit the visual. But I wondered if this man with low standards for the women he dated would find me undatable if he knew my secret. I got the chance to find out during this phone call in the parking lot of my Pilates studio.

Shortly after Ben decided to un-date me, Sandy also called it quits on Mark. The reasons Sandy listed for dumping him, according to Mark, were the same ones I would've used had we been dating and it came time for us to part ways. He was bossy and had advice about everything—even health and fitness, despite that he was unhealthy and unfit. To Sandy's list, I would've added Mark's requirement for face time with his girlfriend. He needed a lot of attention. A hobby would've filled that void, but he seemed to need a lady to occupy his time rather than a self-fulfilling activity. He was like Ben in that respect.

Mark tried his best to console me about Ben's declaration that I no longer call him. Through my car's Bluetooth speaker, he tried to get it through my head that I needed to move on and forget about Ben as an option. Mark was like everyone I knew who had trouble understanding why I couldn't move on.

"He gave me herpes!" I blurted out.

Mark's response was similar to Heather's and Leo's. He hesitated a few seconds to let my words sink in and then replied with an elongated, "Ohhhhh . . ."

After my admission, lunches with Mark began to include open discussions about herpes as well as plenty of jokes about the virus. Nothing about our friendship changed, except now we had another topic to add to the list. The thing I feared most was that, once people knew I was tainted, they would recoil from shaking my hand, hugging, sharing toilets, visiting my house, or allowing me to visit theirs. None of that happened. Heather, Leo, and Mark were better people than me. I might not have been so understanding—just as I was unkind with Jenny, my roommate, years ago—if our roles had been reversed.

Now I could discuss with all three the reasons behind the confounding choices I'd made since my diagnosis. I wasn't just a stupid woman in love making bad choices, like adding Ben to the title of my house or hoping for a reconciliation with a man who wanted nothing to do with me anymore. I was hurt and scared and the motivation behind my stupid decisions was now clear to them.

My search for a house was another example of my chaotic decision-making. If I hadn't had my own real estate license, I don't know that I would've found a realtor who would put up with my house hunting obsession. When it was all said and done and I closed on a house, I'd probably looked online at 500 houses, walked through at least fifty, and submitted offers on five.

The first house I tried to buy was a new two-story, with a blank-slate backyard and a walk-in shower in the master bathroom. It was about two miles from Ben's home. It had RV parking along one side of the house where I imagined Ben could park the camper he talked about getting while we were still together. When he'd talked about the two of us taking camping trips with his kids, my skin crawled at the thought of being in such tight quarters with people who openly disliked me. Now I would've walked sheepishly, with my mouth shut in utter compliance, into the camper if they would've allowed me in.

The market was very competitive at that time and I was outbid. Holding back tears when the seller's realtor called to tell me her client had accepted a better offer, I tried but failed to keep my voice steady and professional. The realtor was sympathetic to me and apologized on behalf of her client.

Friends and family members questioned the logic behind buying a house so close to Ben when I had a whole valley full of living quarters to choose from that were far from my ex-boyfriend and his kids. I justified my choice of locale by explaining, truthfully, that I had searched a large swath of area from within a few miles of my office to areas that were a forty-five-minute drive away. When I explained that I wanted to stay in the area where I'd lived with Ben because that locale fit my lifestyle best, I wasn't lying. I'd liked my easy, fifteen-minute commute to work, and my Pilates studio was just as close. Also, the houses in that area were about twenty years old and had bigger yards than newer places, which tended to have backyards extending just a few feet from the backdoor to the property line. I'd enjoyed taking care of the yard with Ben and I hoped to expand my knowledge and develop a knack for gardening in my own house. In the process, I hoped to grow something better than what I'd grown with him and fantasized he'd someday see what I'd built and be impressed.

There was enough truth behind the motivation I shared with loved ones to covertly leave out the part that living close to Ben would be advantageous once we started seeing each other again.

Lone Mountain was another amenity to add to the list of things I liked about the area. Its name accurately depicts what kind of mountain it was—a single rock that stood alone, unconnected to a range of other mountains. It was circled by a 2.5-mile trail used by people on horses, bikes, or on foot enjoying a somewhat challenging stroll of various elevations. If the walk around the mountain wasn't challenging enough, you could take a strenuous stroll to the top for a beautiful view of the entire Las Vegas Valley. Even though I hadn't used the trail much when I lived by it, I liked the exercise options the trail provided, and I used those options as a reason to explain why I wanted to live in my old neighborhood.

There were expensive houses to the east of the mountain and upper-middle-class homes to the west. In my search for a new place, both sides of the mountain were unobtainable—until a miracle happened. A 2,024-square-foot, two-story house west of Lone Mountain went up for sale and was within my price range. I made an appointment to see it the next day and submitted an offer before the sun set. Two days later, my offer was accepted.

The only problem with my manic search for a house was that Ben hadn't completed his refinance. If I'd been able to use common sense at that time, I would've waited until his financial hurdle cleared me of my obligation to our joint mortgage. Instead, I chose to continue my search in the hope that it would all time out perfectly. This caused me unbelievable anxiety and lots of tears considering the very real fact that my purchase could fall through if he was unable to get his finances in order.

Although I didn't see it at that time, luck was occasionally on my side. While I was still within the forty-five days my contract gave me to complete my own mortgage paperwork, Ben called to tell me his tax return had been accepted and his refinance paperwork was ready for signing. Ben wanted to pay for a mobile notary to meet us at *his* house to complete the paperwork, but I refused to step foot into that house. I imagined his kids standing by to witness as I signed away my house and they looked on in glee. To get my signature, I insisted he would have to come to me at my place of employment.

It was a Saturday in October when he pulled into the parking lot and greeted me with a smile. I was wearing yoga clothes to show off my slim figure. His eyes scanned my body up and down with approval. As we stood face-to-face in the parking lot, he put his left hand on my right hip and told me I looked good. For a guy with a girlfriend, who no longer wanted me to call or text him, that gesture of touching me so intimately angered me. How dare he act like he had permission to touch me when he told me I was no longer welcome to contact him! Would his new girlfriend approve of that touch? I rudely pushed his hand away and all friendliness left his body.

The rest of the transaction was business only. The mobile notary, a non-descript White man in his forties, arrived and the three of us went silently together to my office. During the short trek to the second floor, I whispered to the notary that Ben was an ass, to which the notary made no reply.

I pouted like a baby during the signing, sitting mournfully with my arms crossed with two men who cared not for my feelings and mostly ignored me. My part in the signing was small compared to all the signatures required of Ben to complete his sole ownership of our home. After the signing was done, Ben couldn't get away from me fast enough and refused to have any further conversation with me. I returned alone to my stupid apartment and Ben no doubt returned to *his* house and celebrated my removal from the title by taking his girlfriend and kids out to dinner.

After I closed on my house a few weeks later, I hired a moving company to move my belongings from my apartment to my new house, and I begged my mom to fly to Vegas to help me. None of my friends offered assistance and I didn't have the courage to ask anyone for help. I couldn't take a rejection and felt it was better to rely on my seventy-two-year-old mom than face being told no by people I would've helped move, whether I wanted to or not.

I had a meltdown after a snafu with the moving company almost delayed my move. I found out the day of the move, when the truck and movers failed to arrive at the appointed time, that I wasn't on the schedule. I cried and complained to Mom that nothing was going right for me anymore.

The fear my mom felt for my sanity was obvious in her eyes. I shared her fear. It seemed like God wasn't on my side and I struggled to understand why I was being hammered down so hard by life and Ben wasn't. Was I so wrong that I needed to be corrected so aggressively with one bit of sadness after another? And was Ben so right that he was rewarded with love so soon after our breakup? And his kids could continue on unchecked in their childish, mean ways?

Within an hour of my meltdown, some luck came out of nowhere to change the trajectory of the day. The moving company called to say they had a spare truck and crew ready. By the end of the day, I was moved into my new place, and Mom and I spent the next few days cleaning and putting stuff away. Leo even came over to check things out and help hang a couple shelves in my master bathroom.

Ben could have easily found my new address if he'd wanted to by searching Clark County's online property records database, but I felt the need to text him that information anyway. It wasn't the specific address I was interested in relaying to him; I wanted him to know that he could stop by anytime to see where I was living. I texted him my address with a nice message that he was welcome to come and see my new place at his leisure. He responded by not responding.

I have since learned that no response is a response, even though it's a cop-out and shows a lack of integrity. I continued to listen to podcasts Anisa recommended on going no-contact after a breakup, and I took those messages to heart despite the constant, silent nagging in my mind to reach out to Ben. Little memories would cross my mind of good times we'd shared, and I would fight myself from sending a text to remind him.

Lots of these little memories came up due to the fact I'd bought a house so close to the places where we used to eat or shop. To make matters worse, within a very short time after my move-in, I passed by Ben twice while driving, me in the Cadillac we'd bought together and him in his huge truck. I had no idea if he saw me, but I sure saw him, and I felt stupid because of the nagging feeling in my gut telling me he was never going to want me back, and that I'd bought a home close to him hoping he would.

His truck displayed his business name and phone number on decals stuck to the driver and passenger doors, as well as to the tailgate. When he'd bought this current truck a year earlier, he'd been unable to use the magnets from his previous vehicle because the new truck was plastic and the magnets wouldn't stick. I'd taken one of the magnets to work, used the printer to scan it at a high resolution, and found a local printer to make stickers. Problem solved, thanks to me! I hoped when he traded in his truck in a year that he'd think of me and all the ways I used to help him with his business and ultimately regret his decision to cast me out of his life.

In the meantime, while I waited for him to feel even the smallest amount of regret, I was stuck for at least two years in a house that was now too close for comfort to my ex. If I sold it any sooner than that, I would've had to pay capital gains tax on any profit. I devised a plan to modernize and remodel my house while I lived in it. There was always some kind of remodel project going on in the house Ben and I co-owned and I didn't mind the inconvenience of not being able to use a bathroom for a bit while it was remodeled, or not use the kitchen, or whatever space Ben decided needed updating. I had my real estate license and buying a house every two years and remodeling it for resale could be a nice way to occupy myself and make a little money.

My next house would definitely be further away from Ben to avoid the memories and street encounters that were making me uncomfortable. I gloated at the thought that he might find out that I'd moved and was using the real estate license that he'd wanted me to get for his company's benefit to make money for myself. He would see that I was a smart, independent woman who had adapted to our breakup and moved on.

At least I hoped to have moved on by then.

Chapter 33
Meet at the Bank

In January 2019, six months after my mind took a deep dive into the darkness, the escrow company Ben and I used for the home we owned together closed out our account and sent the remaining money held in escrow, in the form of a check, to me at my new residence. It seemed weird the check followed me to my new place rather than be sent to Ben, the homeowner who remained in the residence the escrow account had covered, but I suppose I was the primary person on our mortgage and legally obligated to receive the remaining funds.

Ben and I both needed to sign the check in order to cash it. He hadn't had any communication with me since the signing at my office, but this was money...he loved money. I thought for sure he'd reply to a text from me, even if the text requested the two of us seeing each other again, because he'd feel entitled to his money.

After three hours, which felt like an eternity, I got Ben's reply: he'd meet me at a specific bank, on a specific date, at a specific time, to cash the check. When the day came, I arrived at the bank first and waited anxiously for him to arrive. When he did, he greeted me as if we were adversaries who needed to be cordial to each other for the purpose of peacefully completing a business transaction. He walked fast toward the bank's entrance and I followed a step or two behind. We entered the bank and stood in line for a short time until it was our turn at the window. There were too many people around to talk while we waited for our turn with a teller. I asked if we could talk outside after the transaction and he agreed. I was angry at his cold manner and did my best to keep my composure.

After we both received our share of cash, we went outside and talked for a short time near my car. I wanted to give Ben the impression that I was over the breakup and had moved on now that I had a house. My goal was to listen without arguing or rehashing any conflict from the past. Our relationship was over and I was going to show him that I was over him.

I managed to show no emotion when he talked about his girlfriend, who he said knew he was at the bank meeting me, until he said Maddie liked her. Within weeks of beginning their relationship, she had taken Maddie for coffee at Starbucks and the two got along famously. I threw my head back in disbelief, holding back my anger that he would throw that in my face. After our breakup, I had suggested meeting with Maddie and her mother at Starbucks to try and make amends, but Ben had refused. The fact that he allowed the new girlfriend to take his baby girl out for a sugary coffee hurt me to the core.

I told him about the two cats I wasted no time in adopting from a shelter after I moved into my house. I got the first cat in December and, when one wasn't enough, I got a second in January. I hoped Ben sensed how important having cats was to me and that his son's fake allergy—which Ben had used as an excuse for us not to get a cat—was one of the causes of our relationship discontent.

He asked me if I was dating and I said yes. I told him about Positive Singles and said, because of that dating site, having herpes wasn't as scary as I thought it would be. He agreed; having herpes was no big deal. His opinion was no doubt true, but my claim that it wasn't scary to me was a bald-faced lie. I was petrified and had no self-esteem, but that wasn't the image I wanted to project to Ben. I wanted him to see that I was single, fearless, and confident, even though I was anything but.

I filled him in on Jeff, a retired rich guy from California who drove a Porsche, who I'd met through Positive Singles. I left out the part that he was fifty-eight years old to my forty-six because I felt his age diminished his other attributes, including his past as an executive for an entertainment company in California, as well as his wealth. Age was one of the reasons I preferred not to date Mark, but Jeff was successful, with herpes, and I made an exception.

Ben asked if we'd had sex and I said yes, which was true. What I left out of the story was that Jeff dumped me shortly afterward because, he said, I was emotionally unavailable.

Jeff was no taller than me and bearded, Jewish, and new to Las Vegas. He'd been living in Florida for several years with his third wife, a woman he described as my age, taller than him, and beautiful. She was an Eastern European immigrant who'd done some modeling in her younger years. She had three teenage kids Jeff got along with and cared for.

Except for the fact Jeff was successful, he wasn't my type. He seemed soft in the sense that I doubted he'd ever handled a power tool, or at least he wouldn't have bothered to try and use one because he could simply pay someone else to do whatever he needed the tool for. He was also too old for me and I worried that being retired would make him too needy and expectant that I'd always be available to hang out with him. But my goal at that time wasn't to find a forever guy; I was looking for someone to help me get over Ben. If I happened to find someone, and whatever romance we started turned into a relationship, I would've been happy with that, but it wasn't long-term I was after.

Jeff and I bonded over the fact that our significant others probably both had herpes and knew it when they'd started dating us. He was stunned when, after dating the Eastern European for a bit, an STD blood test came back positive for HSV2. Jeff had never experienced an outbreak and his soon-to-be-wife claimed the same, although she would experience outbreaks soon after, same as Ben. The Eastern European blamed Jeff for her outbreaks, to which he couldn't deny that maybe he'd given it to her. With her not admitting to any knowledge of carrying the virus prior, same as Ben, there was room for doubt about who gave whom herpes.

Unfortunately, the Eastern European was a hothead who liked to punch Jeff when she was mad. The last straw was when she broke his nose during a fight. His divorce was still fresh and his move to Vegas had only occurred in the previous two or three months. He, too, was looking to quickly move on from his past.

Our first date was a quick coffee meet-and-greet. Our second took place at a Mexican restaurant where we each drank a couple of margaritas and talked for a couple hours. I invited him to my place and we had condomless sex. Immediately after, I felt extreme remorse and disappointment and Jeff could feel it.

Before he left that evening to return to the expensive condo he was renting in a Strip high-rise, I told him I couldn't believe I'd just behaved exactly as I had with the married guy I'd dated briefly, and with Ben, which was to have sex on the second date without condoms. I put myself in danger again despite having been bitten by Ben.

Jeff said he thought I was clean because I'd said I'd been with Ben for three years and hadn't had sex since the breakup. But, I said, I didn't have the same knowledge about his sexual history and had just put myself in the same danger as I had before. I could tell my words hurt him. A man wants to hear that he gave a great performance, not that the woman is full of regret.

I was unsure if I'd ever hear from again, but we talked it out the next morning by phone and seemed to move past my regret and his fear that I was mentally unstable like his third ex-wife. We made plans to get together the following Saturday for dinner and a movie, which ultimately lead us back to his condo. We had a fun night—I enjoyed it.

I left early the next morning without hanging around for breakfast or cuddling. I had wanted to take a bootcamp class that morning and I was determined that, even if I were in a relationship, I was going to keep my independence, which I'd lost while dating Ben. Any new guy I dated was going to have to realize that I had a life and would make my own decisions, so even though Jeff wanted me to hang out with him, I had stuff to do and I was going to do it.

When I hadn't heard from him by the end of the day, I texted him to see what was up. He told me I wasn't emotionally available and that he was moving on. I didn't beg him to give me another shot, and I was only saddened that I'd have to find some other man to help me move on from Ben.

Everything beyond the fact that Jeff had money and that we'd had sex was left out of the tale I spun for Ben. I wanted him to know I'd moved on and, like him, was having sex.

"See, having herpes isn't that bad, is it?" he quipped. He'd said this many times during our relationship.

I replied with a simple "no" to his question. But I was lying, lying, lying. Underneath my tough act lay fear.

He went on to explain that the secret to dating with herpes was to keep your secret until after you'd had sex with the unsuspecting person and felt the two of you were sexually compatible. He said he'd told his new girlfriend only after she'd said she wanted to have condomless sex with him. He assured her he was on medication and "couldn't" pass it on, he said.

I told him that was not true, to which he replied that it was indeed true because his doctor had said so. Based on my research, the chances of passing on the virus while on anti-viral medication is extremely low, at about 5%, but still possible. I didn't believe a doctor would ever have told Ben that his medication absolved him of his status as patient zero, but I told myself to keep my mouth shut because his girlfriend was an adult and could advocate for her own health by talking to her doctor or searching Dr. Google.

To absolve himself even further of his infectious status, he said, "I'm not even sure I have it. I've never been diagnosed."

In utter disbelief I said, "Come on, Ben! I saw it on your dick! You took my medication when you had outbreaks!"

Our conversation was over at that point; he'd had enough of me. Maybe we hugged goodbye, maybe we didn't. I don't remember.

I left that meeting with complete assurance that Ben had given me herpes. I saw myself going through life with a conscience, admitting to potential mates that I was a herpes carrier and setting myself up for rejection. All the while Ben, my gift giver, was content to convince himself he was clean. I saw myself being rejected over and over and Ben feigning innocence when and if the women who walked into his life came down with the condition. I imagined him having the same conversation with them as he'd had with me—they could have just as easily given him the disease as he could have given it to them.

I needed the help of my therapist to sort out the things Ben had said outside the bank. I couldn't understand why Maddie would be kind to his new woman or why he would have condomless sex with me on our first encounter while he gave other lovers, according to his own words, the chance to run.

Jenna, my new therapist, said it was simple. He was lying.

I'd switched from Dan, the old male therapist I'd been seeing, to Jenna, a thirtyish, chubby White woman who I felt had a more current perspective on therapy than Dan. While the old guy seemed to be annoyed by my tears and my inability to get over the fact I was single with herpes, Jenna was much less judgmental and I liked her.

"There's no way a doctor would have provided Ben a prescription for a herpes medication if he hadn't been diagnosed with herpes in the first place," Jenna pointed out.

She also pointed out the likelihood that Maddie had turned into a loving and accepting child to her dad's new love was low. Tigers don't change their stripes, she said, especially when they don't have to. While intellectually I believed what Jenna explained, my irrational brain was hurt by the thought that perhaps Maddie had truly decided on her own to be nice. She might've decided to be nice to *me* while I was involved with her father, and I was hurt to think there was something about me she hated so much that she would become kind only after I left.

Chapter 34
DIY Therapy

Not long after I'd moved into my new house, I realized I didn't feel any more at peace with the circumstances of my life than I had in my apartment. Turns out, my theory that owning a new home would magically fix my depressed brain was complete bunk. I searched for distractions but couldn't bring myself to paint crafts, my former go-to, or finally sit down at my computer and get to writing. Both activities, one a known talent and the other still a dream, required hours of being alone, and nothing sent me into a frenzy of anxiety more than being alone with no plans lined up. Being social quelled my endless sense of FOMO, or fear of missing out on the wonderfully fun lives I was sure everyone else was experiencing, especially Ben and his kids.

Too much time alone with my thoughts would lead to ruminating about the mistakes I'd made during my three years with Ben, as well as the wrongs he and his family had done to me, and my fear of a forever-lonely future. To make matters worse, I believed Ben would find out I was alone and lonely and would gloat in the knowledge that I was a loser with no life. He would hang out in the backyard, lounging in and around the pool that used to be mine, and joke with his family and friends that I should've behaved myself to remain part of his amazing life.

I searched for a way to make my house a place where I could hang out without feeling isolated, without dreading the approaching weekends—especially three-day holiday weekends—

and I found solace in DIY home-improvement projects. The Internet had helped me with information about herpes in my darkest days, and now Google and YouTube were teaching me what I needed to know to therapize myself with updates to my home.

Once I got started with home improvement, I couldn't believe I used to wait weeks and months for Leo to do these kinds of projects when all along, I had the capability to do them myself. For some reason, I thought it took a man to handle power tools, such as the electric drill Leo had used to install shelving in my new master bathroom. I felt silly that, weeks earlier, I'd even asked him for help with such a simple chore. I learned that, with a little nerve and determination, I could easily do the things I'd thought came more easily to men.

I actually had Ben to thank for providing the inspiration to attempt my hand at DIYing. I witnessed him on many occasions accomplishing such tasks as changing out electrical outlets or fixing leaks in our landscaping irrigation. These weren't tasks he performed for his clients. He had guys who could do that, usually Mexicans who were unlicensed and in the country illegally. To explain how he had the knowledge to do these jobs, he would say he watched his Mexicans do it, who learned watching other Mexicans do it. They were regular guys from the street and, if they could do it, Ben said, so could he. Using this same logic, if it were possible for Ben and his Mexicans to learn to do the work by watching others do it, so could I with the help of YouTube. I was right!

Of course, there were some projects out of my grasp, such as tile installation. I hired that job out to get it done quickly, as what would've taken me a year to learn and complete could be done by professionals in a week. Although I had the time to learn how to install tile, having the new flooring in place gave my house a lovely new look and feel, and I was happy to have that feeling sooner rather than later.

When I moved in, most of the floors in my house were covered with a reddish-brown carpet. The only place with no ugly carpet was the kitchen, which had an ugly tile covering of its own. The house had had only one owner in its twenty years of existence, and those people had lived in it as a family until turning it into a rental after moving to the Pacific Northwest. Based on the two small handprints embedded into the concrete patio slab in the backyard, that family was probably just starting out with two small kids when they'd bought the house and probably didn't have extra money to invest in upgrades. The tile and carpet were no doubt the cheapest offered by the builder. I also would've put in the cheapest offerings twenty years earlier, when I was much younger with fewer resources. But I was older now, had a few dollars in the bank, and I wanted style—not Ben's modern style or Leo's lack of it, but décor that was 100 percent mine.

I got a good deal on tile from Floor & Décor, a large store that had just opened a couple miles away. I loved the look of wood and the durability of tile, and my chosen wood-like ceramic tile fit my style perfectly. Years earlier I'd had a similar tile installed in my North Las Vegas house and I still loved the look of it. It had become popular in recent years and I'd noticed it in many of the remodeled and flipped houses I'd seen while I was looking. For this most recent redo, I'd snagged the tile at half-off as part of a grand opening special, spending quite a bit less on flooring than I thought I would.

I'd been to another Floor & Décor branch, in Henderson, many times with Ben as we'd either searched for tile for our house or checked on orders for his clients. I knew he was excited for this new, closer branch to open, and while shopping for my own needs, I secretly hoped I'd run into him. I'd casually tell him I'd found a contractor who was ready to install my tile as soon as I found what I wanted, and then I'd casually walk away with a smile on my face, hoping he'd see how strong and independent I was. And then, of course, he'd realize he missed me and call.

I had my new tile installed throughout the first floor, on the stairs and second floor landing, and in the master bathroom. When the installation was done, the only place the old carpet remained was in the three bedrooms upstairs and in the loft. I would replace that carpet, too, someday, but it didn't offend me as much in the sleeping quarters as it did everywhere else.

Next up, I had the installers put a black-and-gray tile backsplash in the kitchen, and hired a granite installer to replace my white, laminate kitchen countertops with black granite. In my frantic search for a home, I'd come across a kitchen I loved with white cabinets, black stone countertops, and stainless-steel appliances, and I'd made a plan to replicate it. The house with the beautiful kitchen was out of my price range, but I could afford to redo my own kitchen in that style, especially if I manned up and repainted the cabinets myself.

Painting the cabinets would be a perfect task to fill the looming Presidents' Day holiday weekend. The Martin Luther King three-day weekend a month earlier had shown me that I wasn't yet ready to be alone with my thoughts for an extended period of time; I needed to keep busy, and a kitchen project became my link to sanity.

I searched images online for proof that regular people had successfully painted their kitchens. Google and YouTube provided plenty of proof that average Joes like me could modernize their spaces with a little paint, new cabinet hardware, and time investment. I wouldn't even have to strip the old stain and varnish or sand down the surfaces before applying the new paint. I went to Home Depot and found the cabinet paint kit recommended by many DIYers, found the brushes I needed, and set off to keep myself busy over the weekend. By the end of the three days, I had a kitchen that matched the photo of the kitchen I admired.

Next, I bought new stainless-steel appliances to replace the twenty-year-old dishwasher, range, and microwave. The refrigerator was already stainless steel and good enough for me. With my redo complete, every time I walked into my house from the garage, I saw a gorgeous kitchen that made me proud not just for the updates I'd paid for, but for the work I'd done myself. I knew that if Ben saw what I'd accomplished, he'd be impressed with my work and initiative.

In painting the kitchen cabinets, I found out that the secret to DIY projects was to just do it. Get it done. Start and keep moving forward. When self-doubt crept into my mind, as it often did during my home improvement sessions, I would repeat to myself that if Ben could do it, so could I. And I could.

I bought and installed cordless blinds for all my windows downstairs and up, changed out all the smoke detectors, and painted the first-floor walls. I chose a color theme of light griege for most of the walls with a darker griege for accent walls here and there. Gray color schemes appeared to be all the rage based on what I'd seen during my house hunt, especially in newer homes or flips, and would someday be the avocado green of the seventies. I didn't care. I liked the colors I'd selected and had the skills, thanks to my own research and work, to repaint my walls if the colors went out of style or I simply felt the need to change.

While I worked on my DIY projects, I tuned into my YouTube breakup podcasts on my desktop computer and cranked up the volume so I could hear the messages from anywhere in the house. I enjoyed the free advice from mental health professionals about how to recover from a breakup. Initially, most of the experts I listened to were Anisa recommendations, until YouTube's algorithm got a hint of what I liked and started suggesting videos from life coaches and others with guidance on changing your mindset to enjoy everyday life.

I set YouTube to automatically play videos one after another. I would pick the first video, and then YouTube would use its algorithm to select and play other related videos one after another. One of those YouTube suggestions was Dr. Wayne Dyer, a motivational speaker and believer in the Law of Attraction, the belief that you attract positive or negative events into your life through your thoughts.

Ben first introduced me to the Law of Attraction one night in bed during pillow talk. The subject came up over a discussion about vision boards, where you find magazine images depicting the life you want to create for yourself, cut them out and paste them to posterboard. If you'd like to live in a gigantic mansion, for example, you'd find photos of the home that matched your desires, put them on your vision board, and display it in a conspicuous place in your home, such as on the refrigerator. Seeing the life of your dreams every time you walk through the kitchen, as well as believing that one day the vision would come to fruition, puts the wheels in motion for the Universe, or God, to deliver.

At the time I mocked the idea of vision boards as a means to delude yourself into thinking that anything other than hard work and knowing the right people could create the life you want. Ben mocked the idea, as his ex-wife had been a prolific creator of vision boards in her efforts to become a world-famous Tony Robbins wannabe.

Even though he would never have created a vision board of his own, he—unlike me—believed that positive thinking could change the trajectory of a ho-hum life into one of wealth and success.

He often spoke of his ability to think creatively and make life happen for him. This ability, he said, set him apart from most other people, including me, who were rule followers and stuck in straightforward thinking, with no peripheral vision. One of his outside-the-box ideas had been to invite his mother to buy into my house in North Las Vegas. She would've paid $100,000 to become a third owner, and Ben and I would've used that money to invest in something else. My mind only saw fear of becoming the minority owner of the house I had invested in for the past fifteen years and worrying about what would happen if Ben and his mom decided to team up against me for whatever reason. I refused Ben's suggestion to bring in his mother as a co-owner because we didn't need her money, her ownership was unnecessary, and I simply didn't want to.

His outside-the-box thinking, to me, was rooted in fearlessness when it came to investing his and other people's money. It scared me, but I also wanted to be a less aggressive version of him. When he'd suggested I read a book called *The Secret*, which explained the concept that *the secret* to creating a dream life is visualization and positive thinking, I gave the book a shot because Ben believed in it, and so did his ex-wife's family, who were successful real estate investors and lawyers. Maybe, I thought, I could implant some of Ben's creative thinking in my brain if I, too, read that book.

I downloaded the electronic version of the book to my Kindle and made an attempt to read it. I didn't get very far into the novel's pages for the simple reason I didn't buy into it at the time. I had always been a person who saw the glass half full, and this Law of Attraction business depicted in *The Secret* was just too optimistic for my liking. It felt naive to believe that something as simple as visualizing a million dollars in your bank account could ever make it turn into reality. People with million-dollar bank accounts were connected, like Ben was connected to his ex-father-in-law. Ben had no construction experience, and if it weren't for his marriage to Deborah, his father-in-law would never have hired him to handle his construction projects, which lead to Ben gaining experience as a general contractor. Connected people weren't simple, small-town people from Wisconsin who were unlucky enough to contract herpes.

· · · · ● · ● · · · ·

One weekend when I was busy painting my walls downstairs while a Wayne Dyer lecture blasted from my computer, Leo stopped by for a visit to check on the Harley Davidson motorcycle he was storing in my garage. He'd asked me some weeks earlier whether he could store a motorcycle at my place if he were to buy one, and I'd said yes. If this cheap man, who lived like a pauper with a lawn chair for living room furniture, was willing to shell out money on a Harley, the least I could do was let him use extra space in my garage. His only parking option at his condo complex was outdoors in a communal parking area and he feared the bike would be stolen if he left it parked in the open. That motorcycle became a reason for Leo to drop by my place every other weekend to check on it, even though he never rode it. We'd end up in a conversation of some sort and sometimes even go out for dinner. I got company out of the motorcycle/garage deal and that was nice.

The only glitch was that Leo had developed a rather rude habit of coming over unannounced and walking into my house without knocking. That day, due to the high volume of my uplifting podcast, I didn't hear him enter. I was in the middle of painting my stairway and his sudden appearance frightened me. My fear swiftly changed to annoyance as he mocked the lecture on the podcast.

One of the few commonalities we'd shared during our marriage had been a pessimistic view on life. His beliefs apparently hadn't changed, but I was working hard to change mine. My attitude toward the Law of Attraction had changed since Ben and I split. The breakup and his multiple rebuffs had caused my self-esteem to plummet and my outlook on life had turned dismal. It went beyond standard, run-of-the-mill pessimism. I was tired of myself and tired of my thoughts, and had opened up to any idea that could possibly pull me out of my misery. I yearned to believe that my life wasn't going to end in loneliness and despair.

Wayne Dyer shared a humorous anecdote about healing, wherein he said that if he had hemorrhoids and someone convinced him that a chair made of crystals was the solution, he would buy the chair. "Why not?" he said. "I mean, all you have to do is understand something called a placebo." I thought maybe Wayne was on to something. So, I made my first vision board and taped it to my refrigerator.

Chapter 35

Meetup and Men

To inject some energy into my social life, I became a leader of a MeetUp.com singles group and started a friendship group of my own. That way, I always had something to do outside the house on weekends. This normally would've been way out of my comfort zone, but since the Meetup support group had worked out, I wanted to give it a try with other groups. And in truth, becoming a party organizer was partly for myself and partly because I wanted to create a social life Ben would envy.

I daydreamed of the expression on Ben's face when our paths crossed again and, during our chitchat to catch up, I'd tell him about my MeetUp groups and how I was scheduling and hosting events for my new friends. I'd knock his socks off when I'd inform him that approximately 350 Las Vegans had voluntarily joined my group and anywhere from ten to twenty people were attending my dinners and happy hours at various restaurants and bars. His chin would dip and his forehead would wrinkle as he'd raise his eyebrows in surprise. He'd acknowledge that he'd been wrong about me; I *was* social, after all. The company he kept was the issue, not me.

I'd learned that daydreaming was an important part of the Law of Attraction. You must see the end result of your desires to attract the life you want. For example, if your desire is to have a house with a pool, picture yourself sunbathing poolside with a smile on your face as you bask in the glory of owning the home of your dreams. Of course, you must get off your ass, or GOYA, and work toward your goals. But don't waste time wondering and worrying if you're going to get the house with the pool or how you're going to do it. Worry will just push your goals further back because it's a sort of disbelief in yourself and your goals.

My feelings told me that someday Ben was going to knock at my door. Curiosity about what had become of me would get the best of him and he'd come to check. I believed that he was going to become part of my life again even though I couldn't quite reconcile how we could have a relationship when his kids and their dislike for me wouldn't just go away. I chose not to think about that significant obstacle, as it stood in the way of me achieving my dream of reconciling with Ben.

I was focused on the Law of Attraction day in and day out, thinking about Ben, but the problem with it was timing. I knew that the Universe's timeline can be exhaustingly slow. When our paths would cross again was anyone's guess and the Universe's quiet knowing. What if the destiny of our paths crossing didn't happen for years? What was I supposed to do with myself while I waited for the Universe to work my future out? I was bored and lonely and impatient for company.

Advice from online dating coaches was not to put your life on hold while waiting for an ex to come around again. They suggested dating and socializing after a breakup, while also actively engaging in self-improvement work, because life doesn't end when someone decides to walk away from you. Advice from Law of Attraction experts was to see yourself at your wedding with the person you love, but not to worry about how or when you'd get to that destination. I combined the advice of both groups and dated up a storm while I waited for the day when Ben would realize that I was his best option.

I was also open to the idea that maybe Ben wasn't my best option, and to support this idea, I had active dating profiles on Match.com, Facebook dating, and Positive Singles. I hoped to find someone with whom I could laugh and do things with until my real future revealed itself to me. I texted with and met men regularly for a drink, coffee, or a meal to see if there was a spark.

The consensus among women in "my community," as I came to refer to anyone from my herpes group, was that the best approach to dating with herpes was to disclose our status before a face-to-face meeting with a guy. It was better, we all agreed, to avoid investing in someone emotionally who might walk away once he found out about the burden we carried. Since phone conversations aren't my favorite, I disclosed via text using suggested scripts from the Internet. Surprisingly, I found that my luck finding dating options on regular sites was pretty similar with herpes as to when I had dated without.

Despite my original rejection from the Match.com guy who'd wanted to help me get over Ben until he found out I was a leper, I didn't face that type of rejection again. If I got to the point that I was interested enough in a man to pass along my phone number, nine times out of ten he was unfazed by my status. It really flabbergasted me because, if the tables were turned, I would not have been as open-minded as the men who were open-minded about me.

It seemed like every time I went to my weekly therapy visits with Jessica, I had a new guy to tell her about. She listened without showing any sort of judgment on her face. It wasn't until she let it slip that I was trying to make any guy "fit" that I realized she saw error in my ways. When I questioned her on that statement, I could tell by the surprised look on her face that she hadn't meant to vocalize that specific opinion. She also didn't provide much explanation on what she meant. Her words stuck in my mind, though, and made me question what I was doing.

My first experience with therapy had been with a too-thin middle-aged lady who helped me put an action plan in place to finally end my marital misery and file for divorce from Leo. My second therapist, Dan, seemed annoyed by my weepiness at being dumped by a guy who I felt should have done whatever he could to make me happy due to the fact he'd saddled me with the burden of herpes for the rest of my life. And then there was Jessica, who chose the approach of nonjudgmental listening.

I wanted Jessica to tell me what to do, much like my first therapist had done. Jessica hadn't led on at any point prior that my tactic of massive dating may have been harmful to my overall health. I'd listened to many YouTube dating experts who advised taking time to heal after a breakup. They suggested self-improvement work and introspection as just a couple ways to learn and become a stronger person. But I also knew people—including Ben—who'd dated hard after a breakup and ended up in a relationship. He may have met his current girlfriend while in a relationship with me, but he'd found me during a period of heavy dating after his separation and divorce. I also had a coworker, Jonah, who'd dated hard after his second divorce and had found his third wife shortly thereafter by pursuing a ton of women online until one stuck. I just wanted to get over my misery like Ben and Jonah.

Deep down I knew my timing was off. It had taken me four years to feel strong enough to date after my divorce, and my current reason for dating was to force a recovery. I knew I was still messed up, scared, and depressed. My weight was still low and my anxiety high. There were times I'd get tired of the dating game and turn off my profiles for a few weeks and sometimes even up to a month. I was proud to tell

Jessica about these periods of time. I wanted her to express approval for these dating breathers, but I got only her nodding and listening. Ultimately, anxiety and loneliness would get the best of me, and I'd recreate or reactivate profiles that had been deleted or hidden.

While I wanted so badly to be a tough bitch commanding men to earn the right to sleep with me, I was also afraid to scare off any man with potential. If I thought a guy might be boyfriend material, I'd let him decide on our condom usage. I was too invested in seeking validation from men to do otherwise. I needed to prove to myself—but also to Ben—that I was wanted and loveable despite my virus. The quickest and easiest way to be loved, my broken mind had decided, was to stay silent rather than advocate for myself.

I wanted to have self-respect and boundaries. I'd listen to podcasts about how to develop self-respect and mentally note how I was going to set boundaries with the next guy. But I didn't.

Meanwhile, I'd rarely go out with a guy again after sex because I'd find out, while naked and stupid, that he wasn't my type and I had no interest. Each of these occasions led me down a rabbit hole of self-loathing that would end in me determined to break out of the cycle, and I'd establish a plan for handling the next man in a better and more healthy way. But of course, I wouldn't stick to the plan and the self-loathing continued.

Due to my stupid style of dating and fear of inflicting further harm on myself, I'd taken two STD blood tests that had come back negative for both HSV1 and HSV2. How many people have had similar results and thought themselves clear of the virus when, like me, they carried it?

Chapter 36

Getting Weird to Get Better

I placed my mat near a side wall toward the back of the room and sat down cross-legged as I quietly waited for my first kundalini yoga class to start. In my normal hot yoga, Pilates, or boot camp classes, I sought space in front, standing directly before the mirror. My reasons for preferring the front of the room were twofold: to avoid staring at someone else's back the entire class and to protect my water bottle from other people's sweat. This kundalini class was different. There was no mirror and there wouldn't be people sweating all around me from heat and humidity pumped into the room. There would be chanting, movement, meditation, and all kinds of weirdness, and I wanted to be hidden while I attempted to follow along.

I looked around the room at the other attendees—there were about twenty of them—and wondered who they were and what they did for a living. Most of them were middle-aged women, with a smattering of younger women and a few men. Some of them were dressed in normal yoga apparel like I was, and other more seasoned practitioners—both men and women—were covered from head to toe in white linen.

Their heads were wrapped in turbans or beanies and their bodies were hidden behind loose-fitting garments. These were exactly the type of weirdos that would have kept me away from a class like this in the past. They were people I used to consider simple- minded and liberal, people who could easily be persuaded to wear turbans and linen to chase feelings rather than concentrate on learning a trade or skill and earning a respectable living.

But I was broken now and in desperate need of anything that would help soothe my brain. It had been almost a year since my July 2018 breakup and the start of my massive depression. I was still struggling. Jasmin, one of my hot yoga teachers, spoke often of her kundalini yoga classes and encouraged us to give it a try. Kundalini was more for the mind than the body, she said. Jasmin was a beautiful woman with long red hair who was pushing fifty but didn't look it. Her years spent as a professional dancer in shows on the Strip produced a body that could rival any fit twenty-year-old's. She was light-hearted and laughed a lot in her classes, saying, "nobody said you can't laugh in yoga!"

The way Jasmin described kundalini made it sound weird. In fact, she said she and other kundalini teachers jokingly referred to it as "kinda-loony-yoga." But she also made it sound safe, helpful, and maybe even a little intriguing for the peaceful and healing effects she said it had on the mind. She was not too embarrassed or shy to talk about the journey that had led her to yoga to heal her body from years of dancing, followed by a deeper dive into kundalini to heal whatever was going on in her head. When she offered a free kundalini class, I decided to attend and do whatever weirdness everyone else was doing to see what would happen.

Jasmin had hurt my feelings months earlier when she'd told me I was "closed off," meaning guarded and not open to new ideas. I was taken aback that anyone would have that opinion of me. In a room full of people, I would be reserved and quiet and content to let outgoing people dominate the conversation. I wouldn't have been surprised that people misinterpreted my quietness as shy, but I was convinced that closed off did not describe me at all. I was well traveled, educated, crafty, had a live-and-let-live attitude, and unbeknownst to most, had been to a swingers' club!

Jasmin had shared her opinion of my personality upon joining a conversation I was having with Susan, an acquaintance, in the locker room after one of Jasmin's hot yoga classes. During our idle chatter about what was going on in our lives, I mentioned to Susan the trouble I was having deciding whether to rent a room from Nancy or move into an apartment. While Susan and I were going over the pros and cons of my two options, Jasmin walked into the locker room and Susan invited her to give an opinion.

It was just the three of us in the locker room at that time and it seemed a little strange to be opening up to Jasmin about the end of my relationship, the kids who mistreated me, and my homelessness. Our interactions up to that point had been a quick hello or goodbye in passing. She generally appeared to be in a rush when she arrived to teach class or to shower and leave the studio afterward. But she was popular and friendly and, if she wasn't in a hurry coming and going, she was laughing in conversation with a student or two. It wasn't my nature to interject myself in others' conversations or to bother people with a hello or goodbye if they were occupied with others, so I'd quietly pass by on my way to wherever I was going.

Perhaps Jasmin had noticed my solitary ways, which she misconstrued as being "closed off." I had no problem attending any classes on my own; I would quietly lie on my back on my mat and wait for class to start. I engaged in conversation with others around me generally only if they spoke to me first. I had no problem asking other students what kind of weights the instructor wanted us to use, but it wasn't my nature to make small talk for the sake of making small talk. Still, I was friendly with some women at the studio, including Susan.

Maybe Jasmin had noticed my refusal to say "namaste" after a yoga class. It's traditional for the teacher to end class by uttering this word to express gratitude to the students who took the class, and for the students to reciprocate by repeating it back to the teacher. I found the word too new age and hippie for my liking and kept my mouth shut while the other students filled the room with the sound of their namastes.

Maybe she'd also noticed I made a point to keep my hands palm down on my yoga mat when we were instructed by the teacher, at the beginning or end of class, to lie on our backs in savasana, or corpse pose. The teacher would instruct us to keep our palms up to receive energy from the world around us. I was unconvinced that energy could be transferred from the unknown to me through my open palms. To show my unbelief, I kept my palms facing down.

Jasmin's comment about me being closed off came at the end of our conversation just as she was leaving the locker room. I don't remember what advice she gave me about my living situation, but I could not stop thinking that she thought of me in that way. Here was an outsider who didn't know me well but had seen enough to form this opinion about me.

When I took the time to self-reflect and admit all the ways I was guarded and shut myself off from people and new ideas, I could see that Jasmin was right.

· · · **●** · **●** · · ·

Jasmin offered a free kundalini class mid 2019 in honor of a young Pilates and boot camp instructor named Rebecca who had passed away. I'd heard through another student that Rebecca had died at home due to an accident involving alcohol. Rebecca was Susan's daughter.

I'd taken many of Rebecca's fitness classes and liked her teaching style. She was in her late twenties, a short and voluptuous brunette with a sweet personality who worked for an advertising firm and taught fitness classes on the side. I imagined guys who weren't in her league probably fell for her often because she was so nice and sweet, leading men to think her smile was a sign of interest rather than a personality trait she displayed with everyone.

I'd already stepped out of my comfort zone by organizing my own MeetUp group, learning and trying out the Law of Attraction, and listening to Christian sermons I found on YouTube. And now I was sitting cross-legged in a room full of people about to meditate and chant in honor of a wonderful young woman who'd left the Earth far too soon. Nobody would ever have the nerve to call me closed off after this loony yoga!

Just moments before the class was scheduled to start, Jasmin entered the room and sat on her mat on a stage raised about a foot off the floor, front and center of the room. She was dressed head to toe in flowing white linen and her long red hair was invisible inside a turban. She still looked beautiful and smiled at everyone from her perch.

A large gong hung silently behind her from a stand constructed specifically to hold it, with a mallet covered in soft white padding sitting on the floor off to the side. The only gong noise I'd ever heard had been loud and obnoxious; too much for a small room like this. Little rectangle flags, made from tissue paper of several different colors, were strung playfully along the ceiling on strings hung like Christmas lights. The flags reminded me of the strings of red, green, and white flags hanging above Mexican streets during festivals, except the colorful flags in this yoga room weren't patriotic and I didn't know their significance. Maybe they held no meaning and their purpose was only to make the room look festive and happy.

Susan didn't attend this class, which I could totally understand. It was a while before I saw her again at the yoga studio we both attended, and I assumed she needed time to be away from people who reminded her of her daughter's death. Rebecca's brother was present as a representative of the family. It was his first kundalini class, too.

As the class got going with Jasmin leading the students in chants and movements, I followed along with the others as best I could. The words we uttered were ancient, from India, and I had no idea how they translated to English. Jasmin explained the gist of their meaning and what chanting them was supposed to do to us.

It was summer in Las Vegas and the room was comfortably air conditioned. I'd dressed in exercise clothes because I didn't know how athletic this type of yoga would be. It turned out to not be strenuous in the least. With the cool air circulating in the room, I didn't anticipate sweating and figured I'd be able to wear my pants and tank top to my next workout without bothering to wash them.

To my surprise, midway through the hour-long kundalini session, I began to sweat profusely and tears streamed down my face. Since the reason for the class was in memory of a sweet young woman who died too soon, I had a feeling I might be moved to tears at some point, but I was unprepared for the uncontrolled way my body responded. I tried to play it cool and act like I wasn't weirded out. I have no idea how the movements we made, which were mostly performed from a seated position, in coordination with the chanting, caused this effect on me.

I peeked at other people in the room and could see some of them wiping away tears, but I didn't know if they were also perspiring to the same degree as I was. By the time the class had finished, I was 100% intrigued and had already decided I would try another class to see what kind of response my body would conjure up next time. I walked out of that class feeling like something weird had happened to me, but in a good way. I felt purged of some of the toxins making me so heavy with fear and depression, as if I'd really done something good for myself.

I'd gotten hooked on hot yoga several years earlier after taking one yoga class at a studio that offered only Bikram, a ninety-minute set-series of yoga poses practiced in a room heated to 105 degrees and 40 percent humidity. I had a similar feeling after that initial hot yoga class as I had after my first kundalini class. Something weird, but good, had happened to me.

A desire to change up my normal gym exercise routine had led me to try hot yoga years ago. Bikram then led me to expand to other studios that offered Pilates and boot camp in addition to yoga, which had led me to the studio where Jasmin taught, and eventually to kundalini. I had to wonder at the years-long string of events that had guided me toward kundalini one little step at a time. Maybe the Universe really does know what it's doing in arranging our lives with these little coincidences, just as the Law of Attraction says.

Many yoga and Pilates instructors, just before they say namaste, end their classes with an inspirational message to the students. Two themes come up often during those talks, one being the connection between mind and body. Often the trauma and sadness in our minds lead to pains in our body, such as backaches and headaches. Until we fix what's going on in our minds, body pain will persist no matter the amount of medical intervention undertaken.

The second theme is that time and intention heal all wounds. Years can pass by and the hurt inside you will linger unless you put intention into recovering. A person can maintain a certain level of bitterness toward an ex or hurtful life event unless she purposefully intends to rid herself of the bitterness and truly recover. I understood both messages, but I just wasn't open to them until I was ready. I became ready after my mind broke and time wasn't healing me fast enough.

A few days after my initial kundalini class, Jasmin asked me what I thought of my experience. The hot yoga class she was leading had just started and I was one of many students lying flat on my back in the savasana pose, with my eyes closed and head pointing toward the front of the room. My hands were by my side . . . palms up instead of down.

Yoga teachers rarely stand still in class. They walk around the classroom as they demonstrate moves, explain the proper form and the purpose of each pose, and adjust students' arms and legs to achieve the correct position. I felt Jasmin kneel next to me and thought nothing of it. I figured she was going to speak to the class from her crouched position.

"What did you think of kundalini?" She whispered in my ear as quietly as possible.

My body jerked in surprise at the sound of her voice. I quietly whispered back that I liked it, and that I was shocked that it had made me sweat profusely and cry.

"You needed it," Jasmin replied again in a whisper as she nodded confidently. "You should go again," she said as she moved from her crouched position to standing to continue teaching the class.

"I will," I replied. And I meant it.

Chapter 37

Gratitude

I'd recently started listening to Christian preachers on YouTube and was surprised to find myself encouraged by the sermons; as much as my parents tried to instill religiosity in me and my siblings, Christianity had never inspired me. Anisa, a fan of megachurch pastor Joel Osteen, had tried getting me into God while I was with Ben. She'd texted me a link to one of Joel's YouTube sermons, and I remember being annoyed that she thought I'd be interested in it. I politely replied, asking her not to send me religious content because, I guaranteed her, I would never waste time listening to it. Despite this request, after I plunged into a depressive state post-breakup, Anisa again began sending me links to sermons that she believed might help lift me up. Finally, I was ready to listen.

The first Joel Osteen sermon I heard was titled "It's Worth the Wait." Sometimes the things we pray for don't manifest as fast as we'd like because God has put us in a "wait room," Joel explained. You may have a situation in your life that you want to turn around and you've asked for God's help. While it may seem like change is never coming, according to Joel, "If your situation isn't changing, you are. You're getting stronger as you're being prepared." He cited passages from the Bible to make his point that in questionable seasons of our lives, those times when we're in the wait room, maintaining a good attitude and having patience are key. As a person who was struggling to figure out why I'd ended up single with herpes, the idea of being in a wait room while God sorted out my future sounded appealing.

Meanwhile, I discovered the fascinating similarities between Christianity, ancient yoga teachings, and the Law of Attraction. In all three belief systems, followers are urged to live in the present, as ruminating on the past leads to depression, and worrying about future events that may never happen results in anxiety. Other commonalities: tuning into how our words and thoughts play a role in manifesting our futures and knowing the importance of living in gratitude. From each set of teachings, I learned that when your thoughts go dark, you can quickly think of something to be grateful for and reprogram your mind to see the positives in life.

Like attracts like, so letting negative thoughts occupy your mind will only attract more negativity into your life. Feeling gratitude for the lessons you've learned will attract more positive experiences to you. That thinking is too metaphysical for some people, but it felt better to replace negative reflections with positive ones rather than dwelling on shame, embarrassment, and a pessimistic outlook on damned near everything.

All my life, I'd held onto a belief that it was better to be cynical than to allow myself to be hopeful. I thought a negative outlook made me safer and wiser. When something good happened to me, I assumed a negative counter event was waiting around the corner to prove that I was right to be a pessimist. If I stopped to think about the fact that I got herpes after four years of post-divorce celibacy with only my second sexual partner, I could easily believe my own story that bad things always happened to me. It took work and determination to change my mindset from believing dark lurked everywhere to seeing light.

The mental anguish my breakup caused due to my fear of being single with herpes pushed me to search for ways to stop being a defeated and negative woman. The new me wanted to feel optimistic and worthy of love despite the virus I feared would cause even my mom to think I was nasty and dirty. I set my sights on the life I wanted, one of love and acceptance, rather than what I didn't want, rejection and humiliation, and I wrote it all down on paper.

Nancy originally suggested I use journaling as a strategy to refrain from texting and calling Ben. I turned to paper and pen to write letters I'd never send, as well as to vent my misery rather than inundating my friends and family with my constant negativity and woe. I found it comforting to write down thoughts I knew would be considered cuckoo if they'd been spoken from my mouth, and I felt stronger keeping those words locked on the pages of my notebook. Journaling, like therapy, let me share anything without fear of judgment.

Eventually I switched the focus of my journaling from venting my depressive and forlorn thoughts to tracking my gratitude. It made sense to me to focus on the good things in my life rather than believing I was prone to bad luck and unlovable, destined to be forever alone. The switch from pessimism to optimism felt good; I could feel the heaviness of negativity on my brain lift when recognizing and replacing dark thoughts with ones of gratitude. This little shift in thinking made me feel like I had the power to create the life I wanted.

What life did I want? I wanted a good job and to own my own home. Check and check. I wanted loving family and good friends. Check, check. And I wanted to feel good about myself. That was my main focus, a life in which I felt at ease and content. Eventually, I wanted to find someone to be at ease and content with, but that would come later.

The life I wanted included lots of travel. As a young woman, I had backpacked in Europe alone and I had moved to Mexico to teach English all by my lonesome. But I was older now and knew more about the world; no amount of positivity could shake the thought from my mind that some people just want to hurt others and that I could get myself killed as a woman traveling alone. I knew travel was going to happen for me, but when and how were up in the air until, in late 2019, I saw a flyer at my hot yoga studio for a retreat to Costa Rica that one of the instructors was hosting the following spring. That flyer got my head spinning about the possibility of yoga taking me to places all over the world. A subsequent google search verified that yoga retreats exist all over the planet. I decided yoga would be my way to travel with structure, to be in a group while still being alone, without worrying about my safety as a single lady traveling solo.

Yoga! It was something I'd used to stay fit, and now I was using it in ways I'd never imagined, to open my mind and see the world.

Part III - Acceptance

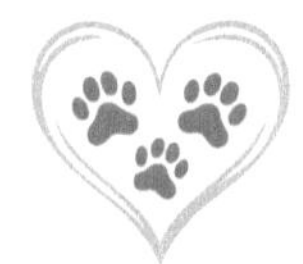

FRS Publishing

Chapter 38

Quarantine

In March 2020, I found out on the same day that, due to Covid-19, my yoga studio was temporarily shutting down and my yoga retreat to Costa Rica was postponed. I'd paid in full for the trip and was sure that these two weeks of quarantining to stop the spread of the virus would be over quickly and life would return to normal soon after. In the meantime, I'd roll with the punches and prepare myself to be stuck at home.

Despite my fear that I'd have anxiety being alone for two solid weeks, I was intrigued at the prospect of experiencing a real-life quarantine. A fan of TV and books about life after a global pandemic, I was interested to see if the stay-at-home order reduced the spread of the virus and if people would maintain civility.

Nevada's governor ordered non-essential businesses to close, which amounted to all brick-and-mortar places of commerce except grocery stores, pharmacies, and home improvement stores. The Las Vegas Strip became a ghost town, with metal crowd barricades and yellow caution tape at casino entrances leaving no room for doubt that all establishments were off limits. What had once been bustling streets with bumper-to-bumper taxi and tourist traffic, and sidewalks full of shoulder-to-shoulder pedestrians, was now empty and dead. Friends on social media posted photos of themselves standing on abandoned sidewalks along Las Vegas Boulevard and wrote about the eerie silence.

I got more experience with quarantine than I expected when what was supposed to be a two-week stay-at-home order turned into two years. After three months, nonessential businesses and casinos re-opened under a mask mandate. However, most Nevada state govern-ment workers remained at home.

Besides the senselessness of it, I learned that quarantine was ex-tremely boring and lonely. The only difference between this lone-liness and what I experienced after Ben kicked me to the curb was that everyone was in the same boat. So, I didn't have the constant nagging feeling, as I'd had the first year post-breakup, that everyone besides me was out doing something amazing. Based on what I saw in online headlines, and from conversations with family and friends, pretty much everyone was feeling lonely and bored.

I'd stopped taking anti-depressants and also quit therapy with Jen-na as talk of quarantine was in the air. Sometimes I didn't have much to discuss anymore during our weekly, hour-long sessions, because I was practicing gratitude and feeling pretty optimistic about my life. The timing felt right to take a break from both therapy and happy pills. Even after Zoom sessions allowed patients to talk to counselors, and when people could go back to face-to-face visits, I didn't feel the need to restart therapy with Jenna or return to anti-depressants. Boredom and loneliness were far different feelings from sadness, and neither required medical intervention.

I also gave up on kinda-loony-yoga. Quarantine required that kun-dalini classes move to an online platform, and it just wasn't the same as attending and chanting with people in person. As a spectator instead of a participant, I got nothing out of the classes from the vantage point of my living room couch. There are some things, at least for me, that do not transfer to the online world, and kundalini was definitely one of them. But I like to think I'd simply had moved on from the need to get weird to get better. I didn't need those classes anymore.

While I could text, talk, or Zoom with family and friends during this period, those first few months when mostly everyone hunkered down at home were brutal. Restaurants and bars were shuttered—there were no lunches, no going out for drinks. I had time, lots of it, and I needed something tangible, activities that were physical, mentally stimulating time killers, and I found my salvation once again in DIY projects.

I bought paint, antiquing medium, and brushes, and then watched YouTube videos about refinishing furniture. I needed a project to throw myself into during my solitary confinement and this one was perfect. When I was done, I'd refinished a TV stand, wall mirror, and bookshelf to match the farmhouse-style kitchen table I'd recently purchased.

As time dragged on, I also painted my upstairs walls to match the downstairs; painted my bathroom vanities gray and added frames around the mirrors; refinished all my doorknobs, hinges, and bathroom lighting fixtures, turning them from silver into bronze; installed new bronze plumbing fixtures in all the bathrooms; replaced torn and tattered window screens; and, as if those projects weren't enough, painted all my floorboards throughout the house a bright white. To complement the work I did myself, I hired a carpet installer to replace the remaining carpet upstairs in the bedrooms, and I bought two comfortable outdoor couches to accommodate the guests I hoped to have over someday for backyard chats and barbeques.

But the best upgrade of all was the installation of a giant walk-in shower in my master bathroom. I hired a company to remove and replace the existing plastic tub and tiny walk-in, prefabricated shower, with a giant shower utilizing leftover floor tile from the floor work I'd done when I first moved in. I'd meant to return the boxes of unused tile but never got around to it. My procrastination worked perfectly because that tile looked beautiful as shower walls. With the addition of this upgraded shower, my house was done.

If my plan had still been to sell after two years and move into another fixer upper, I would've been ready to move ahead at this point. Unfortunately, low interest rates meant housing prices in Las Vegas went crazy during the pandemic. I could've sold my house for way more than I paid for it, but I would've had to blow all that profit on buying something else. Fortunately, I loved where I lived and was content to stay put.

Back in 2018, when I was in the market to buy a place, everyone and their brother advised me to remain living with Nancy or live in an apartment until the housing market tanked. I now felt lucky that I'd listened to my crazy self and purchased a house. I would've gone mental all alone in my apartment, with nothing to do, during two years of work-from-home.

My kitchen table became my workstation to perform my employment duties. I had an unoccupied desk sitting upstairs in my loft that had been meant for crafting, but I considered upstairs too lonely and closed off from the rest of the house. From my first-floor vantage point, I could see through a window at the front of the house and note any life passing by on the sidewalk or street. I could also peer through two larger windows out to the backyard; I would gaze and daydream about what I needed to plant next.

By the grace of God, garden nurseries were deemed essential and were allowed to remain open. Looking out the back window from my workstation, I devised plans to add color and height to my outdoor landscaping, which necessitated trips to the nursery to find suitable plants, flowers, and vines. I was not alone in utilizing my yard to keep busy. The nursery bustled with shoppers who were like me, passing the time keeping their hands busy so their minds didn't go crazy.

I'd always loved landscaping and plants but had never taken the time to learn how to garden in Las Vegas' extreme summers. Turns out, I could simply join local gardeners in social media groups and go to local nurseries to ask about plants that thrived in the heat! Looking out the window to the backyard made me regret not turning my North Las Vegas property into a happy place, leaving the yard vacant and untouched. But I also had to admit that back then, the timing wasn't right. A key part of gardening in Vegas is irrigation, and I didn't learn about that until I was with Ben and observed the ease with which he fixed leaks on existing irrigation lines and installed new ones. I thought all of that would be too complex for me, but I saw with my own eyes, watching Ben, that it wasn't. I became a pro at adding drip lines and making repairs, and as a result, my yard flourished. Despite the solitary nature of my Covid existence, I was thankful for the timing of my life's events, that I'd gained so much knowledge about gardening—and now had a chance to use it.

One practice in the Law of Attraction is to believe that life is happening *FOR* you, not *TO* you. It's up to you to see the lesson in all your experiences and know that you are exactly where you are supposed to be at any moment in time. My ego wouldn't completely let me feel that herpes had happened *for me*, not *to me*, but I could look at other aspects of my life and see how life had happened for me. I loved my house—it had more space than my North Las Vegas place and was closer to everything. I'd transformed the interior of my house myself, turning it into an oasis, a place I wanted to spend time. None of that would've happened had I not met and dated Ben—I might've remained in my old house, with its ho-hum décor and ugly backyard.

This house turned out to be the perfect place for me to live during the years of working from home.

While my yoga and Pilates studio was forced to stay closed, I discovered the joy of walking and considered myself lucky to live in an urban area that provided two mountain trails not far from my front door. There were the paths up and around Lone Mountain, and not long after quarantine started, I discovered an unnamed four-mile loop just a short drive down the road. Those four miles turned to six if I walked it from my home.

Walking had been something I engaged in occasionally when Ben wanted to walk around Lone Mountain or the neighborhood for a little exercise, but I didn't consider it a true form of exertion. I felt that if I weren't jogging or in a fitness or hot yoga class, I wouldn't get good exercise. Now, every day, I put my earbuds in, tuned into a positive podcast on YouTube, and walked.

Afternoon strolls became a way to break up the monotony of hour after hour alone, seeing coworkers in online meetings or communicating by email or text. I spent so much time outside walking that my shoulders turned a deep tan and my medium blonde hair turned light blonde from the sun. I'd never gotten so much outdoor time in all my years in Nevada.

Even after my exercise studio reopened, I kept on walking. I'd take a fitness class in the morning and then hit a trail in the afternoon, when it was too hot for most people to be outside. Being alone on a trail didn't bother me one bit. It was nice to have it to myself, with just me, my podcasts, and the sun.

· · · · ● · ● · · · ·

When I'd work at the kitchen table, my eyes would wander often toward my backyard, where daydream after daydream waited for me. The Law of Attraction says daydreaming tells the Universe the life you want. Similarly, Christianity says not to be ashamed of big prayers and to ask big.

At this point, it had been two years since Ben and I had parted ways. Online dating had been a mixed bag, and while I was no longer awash in anxiety over our split, I still missed him. I still thought about him. What I wanted, at a minimum, was for Ben to check on me, and that's what I asked for.

I wasn't sure what I wanted from Ben after his reappearance in my life. In my daydream, I saw him showing up on my doorstep unexpectedly. I led him around my house to point out all that I'd done to it since I moved in. We eventually moved to the couches in my backyard to enjoy a coffee together, as we'd done so many times during our relationship, and we talked. He admitted that he'd made a mistake dismissing me and that he wanted me back. At that point, the daydream stopped. I was unsure if I wanted anything more than just being recognized and wanted, because I sure didn't want to try and fit myself back into his dysfunction.

I'd reached out to him early in the pandemic, inspired by a neighbor who'd passed along her phone number to me through another neighbor just in case something happened and we needed to take care of each other. Surely Ben, who'd wanted to retire with me not even two years earlier, would care about my wellbeing and want to know how I was doing.

I thought about texting him a greeting but settled on an email based on the likelihood that he'd probably blocked my number. I typed up a short paragraph to tell him that I was well and let him know how I was passing my time during quarantine. I added that I was practicing forgiveness and that I held no ill will toward him, his kids, or myself, for that matter, for what happened to bring about our demise. I didn't mention herpes and the devastation that I felt was his fault. I thought my email was a sweet and kind message that showed no indication of the begging woman I'd been when our relationship ended. I thought surely he would reply to this normal person who just wanted to wish him well.

He didn't.

As the pandemic stretched on for months and work-from-home became an endless way of life, I found the isolation rather crazy-making. I did have a social life—my "community" group started meeting for a monthly brunch once restaurants reopened, and I met regularly with "regular" comrades I'd made in my friendship group. But with zero human contact during the workdays, quiet nights at home were filled with loneliness and persistent thoughts that I needed companionship. There were only so many shows to binge-watch, only so many podcasts to listen to. So, I searched for excuses and looked for signs from the Universe to reach out to people, hoping to curtail the amount of time I spent in solitude.

One day I saw an article about how a man died from eating too much black licorice—Ben's favorite—and convinced myself that it was my sign from the Universe to contact him again as a friendly gesture. It had been a couple months since I'd emailed him and impulsively, I took another crack at it. I texted the article with a short note saying that he better be careful because licorice could be deadly. I probably used a smiley-face emoji to let him know I was joking.

Again, he didn't reply.

It hadn't yet sunk in that loneliness was driving me to make questionable choices. Eventually, however, I had no other option but to accept that Ben's silence *was* the actual sign from the Universe. Whether or not I was blocked from his phone didn't matter; the licorice text had to be my last attempt to communicate with this person who had no interest in my extended olive branch.

Accepting this message from the Universe also meant no more peeking at his ex-wife's social media. Ben used Facebook to keep up with other people's lives and to wish his friends happy birthday, but he didn't do any postings of any kind about his life or business. By looking at Deborah's page, though, I could guess what was happening in Ben's house. Her attempt at being a motivational speaker apparently meant every moment of her and her kids' lives had to be on display on social media, including her daughter's apparent transition into either a butch lesbian or a trans man. I asked Jessica if that's why that girl had been so mean to me—she was confused and angry and took it out on me. All Jessica could say was, "possibly." Whatever the case, I banned myself from social media snooping and have no idea what has become of anyone in that family.

· · · · ● · ● · · · ·

In recent months, I'd been on the dating apps but hadn't been attracted to anyone. I had profiles on two sites— Positive Singles to meet my "kind," and Match.com to see what the non-herpes world had to offer. At one point, I deleted my Positive Singles profile and decided to do a little social experiment with my Match profile for the few weeks remaining on my subscription; it would be for my own amusement and because I had nothing to lose.

I got the idea for this experiment from a man on a Facebook herpes singles group. In his Match.com description about himself, he'd posted that he had HSV2, detailed how he got it, and recounted how it affected his life, and how it may—or may not—affect the woman he dates. He said he was pleasantly surprised at the positive responses he got. *What the heck,* I thought, I'll try it too.

By this point I'd shared my status with a few friends and had developed friendships with several people from my herpes group. I liked that I could talk openly about my status with these people and that they didn't treat me like a dirty whore who should be shamed into silence. Some in the group were afraid for anyone to know and vowed to forever keep their silence. Others had developed an opinion similar to mine: we didn't see what the big deal was about a herpes diagnosis and were unbothered by the thought of being found out by those closest to us.

Still, I hadn't told my family about my diagnosis, and posting my status in the open on Match could lead to it being seen by the wrong person, who'd blab my condition to the world. But I also didn't care and perhaps hoped a bit that I would be outed. It would've been a relief to no longer have the secret, and it would've helped my family understand some of the decisions I'd made over the past few years.

My Match profile led to message exchanges with a few different guys, but no actual meetups with any. I got close to actually going on a date with one guy, but he texted and called at all hours of the day and night and it turned me off. I was lonely and wanted company, but I didn't want to be smothered. I told that guy I wasn't right for him. My mind had moved beyond the need to find validation through a relationship at that point. My Match subscription expired and I deleted my profile and was happy about it.

In the meantime, I set my sights on writing. The Law of Attraction preaches that to obtain a goal, you must talk about yourself as if you'd already achieved it. So instead of saying, "I hope to be a writer someday," you say, "I am a writer," even if you hadn't actually gotten around to writing anything yet. With that thinking in mind, I decided to open up to my friends Heather and Nancy about my writing attempts and the story ideas I was working on. Rather than being the cheerleaders I thought they'd be, I learned it was it was better to keep my writing goals secret.

At dinner one evening with Heather and Nancy, I told them about an idea I had for a novel centering around a post-pandemic scenario. To my surprise, Nancy lectured me on the many reasons why a book based on a pandemic was an unsuitable topic for me. She said it would work for her sons, maybe, but not for me. I was stunned into silence as she explained why any of her three sons would be perfect authors of such a novel due to their love of science fiction. I, however, was unqualified, despite my love of zombie tales.

Alone with Heather on another occasion, I told her maybe my first book should be autobiographical about my experience of revolving my life around the fact that I had herpes, the subsequent depression that resulted when that way of living failed, and the way I worked myself out of it. Heather thought that idea was horrible. She didn't doubt my ability to write on the subject; rather, she said nothing good could come from reliving the experience while I wrote about it.

Luckily, I'd come upon Christian sermons and self-help teachings that advised me to keep my goals secret for the simple fact that some people, for whatever reason, shit on your dreams. Christian teachings say the devil works through negative people and self-doubt to convince you to hate life and live unfulfilled. Self-help aficionados teach that people may poo-poo your dreams to try and protect you from failure. Whatever the case, both schools of thought advocate for silence, and I learned to be good at it while moving forward.

Chapter 39

Walking with Freddie

While I worked from home or worked on my book, I took breaks to walk with my dog. Freddie has been one of the biggest—maybe even *the* biggest—game changers in my life. During quarantine, after I became an avid walker, I'd note all the people out walking with their dogs while I walked alone. They made me feel envious, so I got myself a walking buddy. Freddie has been the best decision I've ever made. EVER.

Before I got Freddie, I dipped my toe into the water by fostering a dog. I did this so that I could 1) help an animal in need and 2) see what urban dog ownership entailed. Up to then, I'd only known what it was like to have a dog in the country, during my rural Wisconsin childhood, and as an adult, I'd only had cats. I was used to cats' independence; if left for a few days, they managed to care of themselves without destroying furniture or defecating all over the house.

I was put in charge of a six-month-old black and white Jack Russell baby boy with a broken front leg. My time with him was short-lived, and we were unable to take walks together due to his injury, but I fell in love with the companionship and love I got from that dog. Unfortunately, the rescue had other plans for him and I couldn't keep him.

Because shelters and rescues were nearly empty due to stay-at-home workers like me looking for company, I turned to craigslist.com and found a tan and white ten-month-old Toy Fox Terrier, which looked an awful lot like a Jack Russell, with a $300 re-homing fee, and immediately emailed the advertiser for more information. That evening, I agreed to meet the little dog's owner, Chad, at a park near his home. I put the $300 in my purse knowing there was no way I could go see the dog without taking him home with me.

Chad was a limo driver on the Strip and had been out of work due to quarantine. He and his wife, who was a state worker like me, had two small daughters. Perhaps spending so much time together quarantining was too much for the family. Chad said he and his wife were separating and he couldn't take the dog with him wherever he was going. The wife simply didn't want him. Chad repeated a few times that she was Mexican and that Mexicans don't like animals in the house. I didn't mention that I'd been married to a Mexican who had no problem with our house cats. I handed Chad my money without dickering over the price, and he handed me my new best friend.

Almost as an afterthought, as I was loading my dog and his crate into my car, I asked for his name. Chad replied that it was Spot. After I got Spot home, I texted photos to family and called my sister to discuss his name, which somehow didn't fit. Doreen told me her plan to adopt a little dog later in life, during retirement, and name him Freddie, after the singer Freddie Mercury, with whom she had become infatuated after watching the movie *Bohemian Rhapsody*. She'd known nothing about the man prior to seeing the movie and felt an intense sympathy for him afterward. That name was perfect for my new dog and I stole it, with Doreen's permission, of course.

The morning of our second day together, Freddie and I started walking and we haven't stopped since. Because of Freddie and being outside passing through the streets in my community, I've met several neighbors who've turned into friends. Las Vegas has a reputation for being a cold city with neighbors living next to each other in anonymity and silence. I used to be one of those people who was happy to avoid and be avoided by neighbors. What a mistake I'd made in my previous twenty-three years in this town. It's a good feeling to know my neighbors and I'm thankful to Freddie for bringing me out of my shell.

Freddie is seventeen pounds of love and energy, and he is the love of my life. I used to think little dogs were a bit useless for their lack of ability to protect and hunt. But now I know the true purpose of a little dog is to be a companion, a sidekick, and they are perfect at it! Freddie is by my side day and night, and he has helped immensely with my anxiety about being alone. I will honor him always with love and a comfortable life for the love and comfort he has brought to mine. I would recommend everybody get a dog!

Chapter 40
I Got a Story

In the fall of 2020, I received a text from Nick, a man I used to work with at the building department. He'd been a good friend of mine during the four years we were coworkers, but I hadn't been in contact with him for several years.

He had a reputation as being a ladies' man, which he cultivated by openly talking about his conquests with everyone, including me. I had an office job and he was a building inspector who spent most of his workday in the field. I looked forward to the end of the day when he'd come back to headquarters with the rest of the inspectors to finish their day completing paperwork. He'd stop by my office and tell me stories. We laughed a lot, and I was sure that he'd be fun to date.

Nick was in his early forties and balding, handsome but not devastatingly good-looking. He had a boldness, though, like Ben, that I found so so so attractive! But for the fact that I was married, I would have let Nick make me one of his stories.

Our contact with each other dwindled after he was laid off during the Great Recession and I took a job with the state. I was surprised he still had my number because I had long since deleted his. Nick said he'd texted me to say hello early on in my relationship with Ben, but received no reply. I don't remember ignoring his text, but logically it seems that I probably ghosted him because I'd turned up with herpes and decided to put all my attention into Ben.

Nick had seen my Match.com profile, but he kept this knowledge to himself as we reconnected, and our friendship returned to what it had been. This time, however, we weren't just coworkers who saw each other at the office, went to lunch, and texted on occasion. We now talked on the phone, took walks together around "my mountain," as I referred to Lone Mountain, and hung out at his house or mine. His address hadn't changed since we met, but because mine had, we were only a ten-minute drive apart.

Nick said that while he was hesitant to date me for fear of ruining our friendship, he was willing to take a risk. He commented on several occasions that he'd like to make our relationship romantic. I had every desire to do just that but was afraid of being rejected and so avoided the topic. I didn't want to tell him I had herpes and maybe put a damper on the chemistry we had going. But eventually, I told him my secret during a phone conversation after he asked if my reluctance to date him was because of being hurt by Ben. It was a make-or-break moment, so I told him my true trauma was herpes.

"I know," he replied. "I saw your Match profile. Don't put that shit on the Internet!"

After that phone conversation, I was sure Nick was heaven-sent and that my dating life was over. I could see no other reason why God would bring him back into my life other than that he was destined to be my forever man. Unfortunately, it turned out he was nothing like the character he portrayed himself to be while we were coworkers. Rather than being a lifelong bachelor due to fierce independence, he was full of fears and insecurities and rather hard to get along with, like my ex-husband. He lived in the past and was angered and depressed often by memories. He also thought every ache or pain he felt was proof that he was dying.

Nick's elderly Greek father lived with him, and Nick spent more time alternately hating his dad and trying to please him than trying to be my boyfriend. Nick's parents' divorce when he was twelve had affected him deeply, and he'd modeled his younger years after his "philandering" dad—his word to describe his father, not mine. His daddy issues reminded me of Leo's issues with his father, which probably made me feel a sense of familiarity with a father/son dynamic that should have caused me to run in the opposite direction.

Over the course of four years, we split regularly and were single more than we were together. We were two damaged people who cared for each other but couldn't figure out how to be normal. After each breakup, I'd tell myself to take time to be alone and heal before making any decisions on how to move forward with my dating life. Nick would swing back around just as I was starting to feel lonely and he'd win me back with a laugh. Sometimes I would seek him out and we'd be on again. The back and forth, in and out, bothered me, and it didn't. Eventually—maybe a bit too slowly—I chose myself over the relationship.

I wasn't crushed when our attempts at dating ended and my self-esteem didn't plummet. This was a change from my pattern in the first few years post-herpes, including with Ben, when I was often loyal to men who didn't deserve it. Back then, if someone was willing to give me time and attention, even if it was poisonous to my life, I would take it. My self-esteem only increased as I realized that breakups are something to be grateful for. Nick and I had our time together, and if he wasn't the one for me, that means the right guy is still out there and I'm excited to meet him. To Nick I will forever be grateful for taking me out of the dating field for a while.

· · · ● · ● ● · · ·

At this point, ten years have passed since my herpes diagnosis and seven since Ben and I broke up. I'm still in the same house. I love where I live and what I did to make the house mine. I love my yard, my neighbors, and my mountain trails. I'm living exactly where I'm supposed to be at the moment and that knowledge makes me grateful.

The process of healing takes time and intention. Years could have gone by and been wasted, with no recovery, if I hadn't made the effort to seek help and to change. At different periods during the past years, I'd feel as if I'd healed, but after more time passed, I'd realize I was feeling even better, and that before, I hadn't been as healed as I'd thought. Healing is an interesting process and worth the effort to not wake up every day feeling bitter and pessimistic.

It's obvious from the themes of Christian sermons, the Law of Attraction, and self-help gurus that many people have walked your path before you, whatever that path is. Depression has been around for eons, as has overall human confusion. I was embarrassed at how broken I was after my relationship with Ben ended—but I also came to see that so many people have suffered in similar ways to me. If they hadn't, there wouldn't be advice on how to overcome it. That advice is out there—much of it for free—for anyone who wants to take the time to listen to or read it. It's on YouTube, social media, and in books.

I'm not advocating for any one speaker or philosophy—my advocacy is for being open to messages that resonate. Maybe the Law of Attraction isn't for everyone, or kundalini, or religious teachings, for that matter. They worked for me. But my interest in all three has also changed as I've changed. I rarely listen to Law of Attraction podcasts anymore, and I haven't taken a kundalini class since quarantine, but my interest in Christianity has grown. I went in search of a church not too long ago, and after trying out several, I found one I like and I attend regularly. I enjoy learning about the Bible through Christian sermons and I'm grateful my mind is open to receive.

I am healed from the trauma of having herpes. Everybody has some sort of pain they're dealing with. I hope herpes isn't the source of that pain because it's really nothing to beat yourself up about. It's a rash. Precautions can be taken to not spread it to others, and so many people know that.

You may not understand the suffering you've been through, but if God thought you couldn't handle it, he wouldn't have put you through it. Take the hand you've been dealt and deal with it. Ignoring your trauma just puts you in a place you don't belong—I know that from experience. I was willing to give up the life I wanted to follow Ben around just so I wouldn't have to face life alone.

Speaking of Ben, I do have a story to tell about running into him. It didn't happen during the pandemic like in my daydream. It happened in the spring of 2022, at a plant nursery, two years after quarantine and more than a year after my last reach-out attempt. Deep down, I had a feeling that I'd run into him at a store or restaurant, rather than seeing him when he visited me at my house, as in my daydream.

When God put us in the same place at the same time, I didn't recognize him. Freddie and I had just entered the outdoor section of the nursery when I saw a couple with large, wheelbarrow-like carts coming toward us, headed for the indoor section and checkout. I stepped aside and into a row of plants to allow the woman, a middle-aged Asian lady, and her White fella to pass. Her cart was empty and his held only a few plants. I wondered why they were hanging onto such large carts when they apparently hadn't found what they were looking for. Especially her. She could have left her empty cart outside for someone who really needed it.

I looked at the lady, ready to offer her a smile as she passed by. I was a little surprised that she ignored me, not even glancing my way, when Freddie and I had been kind enough to step aside to let her pass. Behind her I noticed her tall partner beaming with a smile and I thought, *well at least the guy she's with is nice.*

With a huge smile plastered on his face, the guy said, "Hey!"

It was Ben. He was wearing sunglasses, a fleece sweatshirt he'd bought on one of our Costco shopping trips, and black track pants. His hair and face looked a little greasy, as if he hadn't showered.

"Oh!...Hey," I said in reply. It was all my mind could register to say. I was taken by surprise that Ben was standing almost directly in front of me. You'd think that I would've sensed his presence and recognized him right away. But if he'd passed by me without smiling or saying a word, I'm sure I would've given him no more than a glance, and we might have crossed paths with no further recognition.

"You got a dog!" he stated rather happily as he nodded his head toward my best friend.

"Yes," I replied matter-of-factly as Freddie and I moved back onto the sidewalk, just a few feet away from him, continuing toward the plants I'd come to the store to see.

"What happened to cats?" He'd stopped walking and started to set his cart down, as if he intended to have a conversation.

"I still have one," I said over my shoulder as I kept walking. I could've stopped and explained that one cat got out my new doggy door and never came back, but I had no desire to share any information with him.

"Oh, you still have one," he repeated, looking a little confused that I'd kept walking and wasn't going to engage in conversation. He shrugged his shoulders and turned back toward his lady friend, who'd stopped and was watching us. They continued on their way, and I continued on mine in the opposite direction.

At one point during our relationship, he'd told me that if we broke up, he'd like to date an Asian woman because, he said, they were docile and man-pleasing. From what I could tell, he'd put his wish out into the Universe and the Universe brought her to him. I had no idea if she was the original woman he'd started dating while we were breaking up or someone who came later. That information was no concern of mine.

I usually didn't shower before my typical morning trips to the garden center because I'd end up sweaty from the yard work that would occur after. However, for some reason I'd felt prompted to clean up that morning. My weight was pretty much back to normal at that point, but I was put together, happily shopping for plants with my dog. Except for the fact I was presentable during this chance encounter with Ben, not much else resembled the daydream encounter I'd, at one time, hoped to manifest.

After I found the plant I wanted and checked out, I carried it out to the car with Freddie on the leash, trotting next to me. I got into the driver's seat and paused for a moment. What did I feel? Other than a small modicum of satisfaction in having looked presentable, I felt... nothing. No excitement, no giddiness. No wondering whether I should follow up my encounter with a text or imagining that Ben might text me. And then a wave came over me—a wave of extreme happiness. I felt zilch for that man. Finally.

I used to wonder what Ben was telling people about me and our failed relationship. I'm pretty sure he said I wasn't social enough for him and that I wasn't motherly enough for his kids. He was absolutely right. He wanted a woman who would dutifully give herself to tending to him and his kids and happily host dinner parties. He wanted someone who felt the obligation to be what he wanted.

While with Ben, I revolved my existence around the fact I had herpes. I'd shoehorned myself into the life I was living, and nothing felt right about it. The more I tried to talk myself into accepting my fate and being someone I wasn't, the sadder and angrier I got. I based my future on getting through life with herpes by trying to fit into a family and household where I didn't belong, rather than making *my* future fit *me*, and I was miserable.

I used to think that the devil was working through Maddie. I know now that God was working through her. I didn't have the courage to leave a situation that wasn't good for me, so God made it impossible for me to stay. I was going to give up my dream of being a writer just so I wouldn't have to face the fact that I had herpes. Through that kid, God made me face my fears and be who I was put on this Earth to be. I wasn't meant to be Ben's girlfriend. I was meant to be a writer.

Writing involves the same kind of attitude as DIY projects—just do it. Get it done. Keep moving forward. If others can do it, so can I. It took herpes and a near-mental breakdown to get me to finally pursue what I was meant to do. Herpes didn't happen *to me*, it happened *for me*. From herpes I got a story, and for this story I will be forever grateful.

I stopped taking Zika pills at least four years ago and have not experienced a second outbreak. My body has always been strong—I rarely get sick and I didn't get Covid. Herpes had always been more of a mental virus for me than physical. Not anymore.

My time as a civil servant will come to an end before the decade is over and I'm looking into fostering children and beekeeping while I continue writing. I also want to do more with dogs—I have three now. I don't know what that looks like; maybe I'll start a doggy daycare with my foster kids. Whatever the case, I'm optimistic about the future and I'm grateful for that!

As for other aspects of my life—especially romance—I'm once again in the wait room, celibate, and I'm fine with that. I will not force what isn't meant for me. I'm comfortable with who I am, and I look forward to the day I walk out of the wait room holding hands with my partner. The man I walk with will have a story too and I am excited to hear it.

Thank you.

The End

About the author

Dawn Dravir is a bureaucrat by profession, cheesehead by birth and Las Vegan by choice. Born in Wisconsin amid the snowy landscapes and football fanaticism of America's Dairyland—where cheese curds are practically a food group and family life meant squeezing six people into a three-bedroom home with just one bathroom—Dawn grew up immersed in the hearty, no-nonsense spirit of the region. Her early years shaped her grounded perspective, from cheering on the Packers to appreciating the simple chaos of shared spaces.

Armed with a bachelor's degree in English, Dawn writes about midlife, mistakes, cautionary tales, and dogs. She finds solace and joy in daily strolls with her furry companions, Freddie, Ralphie and Sparky, often capturing the magic of Las Vegas sunrises that paint the sky in hues of burnt orange, purple and pink over the Strip's distant glow.

From her humble Wisconsin beginnings to building a purposeful life in Vegas, Dawn embodies the American dream of starting over: practical, passionate, and always up for a good dog walk at sunrise.